Praise for *Seeds of Sisterhood*

"Seeds of Sisterhood is a transformative guide that not only demystifies hormone health but also offers practical, compassionate solutions to support women on their wellness journey. Melissa seamlessly blends the science of functional nutrition, EFT tapping, and the time-honoured practice of seed cycling, empowering readers to reclaim balance and vitality. Her deep understanding of women's health and the power of community shines through every page, making this a must-read for anyone seeking natural solutions to hormone balance and overall well-being."

— *Steph Lowe, Nutritionist, founder of The Natural Nutritionist*

"Melissa has created a powerful resource for women seeking to balance their hormones naturally. 'Seeds of Sisterhood' weaves functional nutrition and emotional healing practices with ancient wisdom, offering readers a holistic path to reclaiming their body's innate rhythm and vitality."

— *Amanda Trieger, (B.Nat, NHAA, SCU, SW Glad, EL) Lead Naturopath at Naturopathic Womancraft Clinic, Trainer for Health Professionals, Vaginal Microbiome Specialist, Pre & Post-partum Doula*

"Melissa Kovacevic beautifully weaves together the transformative power of seed cycling, functional nutrition, and EFT tapping, integrating ancient wisdom to the now and giving women an empowering perspective to gaining natural hormone balance."

- *Nat Kringoudis, The Hormone Revolutionist, Women's Health Practitioner, 2 x Best Selling Author.*

"This book offers a holistic view of hormonal support for women of all ages, no matter where they are in their reproductive journey. It empowers women to deeply understand and work with their bodies, offering a new approach to reproductive health that goes beyond band-aid solutions. The Seeds of Sisterhood supports women to embrace the power of their cycle whilst finding the strength in sisterhood along the way. Whether you're a mother, daughter, aunty or friend, I believe this book should be shared with every woman in your life."

- *Sarina Coventry, Nutritionist (BHSc) & Clinical EFT Tapping Practitioner*

"In Seeds of Sisterhood, Melissa uncovers an essential link between the mind and body, weaving together the roles of food, emotions, and stress in a way that is both elegant and concise. She reframes food as not just nourishment, but as medicine, and explores how our emotions and beliefs about our bodies can profoundly affect our overall health.

What stands out is how Melissa takes us on a journey back to nature. She gently guides us to tap (literally and figuratively) into the innate wisdom of our bodies. In a world flooded with marketing messages competing for our attention—and our dollars—Melissa's message is a breath of fresh air, offering clarity and simplicity. She understands the overwhelming challenges women face just to maintain health, let alone recover from illness or disease, and she eloquently explains the historical and cultural contributors to this struggle, from societal pressures on appearance to the complexities of social and cultural eating.

One of the most valuable aspects of this book is her approach. Melissa shares helpful advice and exercises in a friendly, informed tone, never prescriptive. Her respect for science adds credibility, but she doesn't blindly follow it—acknowledging that true science evolves through continuous observation, questioning, and experimentation. This makes her insights even more trustworthy. A beautiful and empowering book that every woman should read."

– Naomi Janzen, Evidence Based (EBEFT) Accredited Advanced Practitioner and EFT International Master Trainer

"Seeds of Sisterhood is a richly practical, evidence-based and yet wisdom-filled guide for the woman reclaiming her hormone health and seeking to heal her symptoms naturally at the root cause level. Weaving knowledge and traditional wisdom from global cultures together with modern science, holistic wellbeing practices to explore at home and nourishing recipes, this is a highly-recommended empowering, insightful and useful resource for every family bookshelf that supports the menstrual life cycle from menarche to menopause."

–Charlotte Pointeaux, Wild Feminine Embodiment Coach and Priestess, Founder: First Moon Circle School

Seeds of Sisterhood

*Functional Nutrition, EFT Tapping
and Seed Cycling for Natural Hormone Balance*

First Edition

Copyright © 2024 by Melissa Kovacevic

All rights reserved.

No part of this book may be reproduced, distributed, or transmitted in any form or by any means, including photocopying, recording, or other electronic or mechanical methods, without the prior written permission of the publisher, except in the case of brief quotations embodied in critical reviews and certain other non-commercial uses permitted by copyright law.

Book Cover Design by Jon Shirley
Photography Back Cover by Marina Lustica
Editors Mira Lustica, Samantha Mears

ISBN: 978-0-646-70287-2

Published by Melissa Kovacevic via Amazon Kindle Direct Publishing

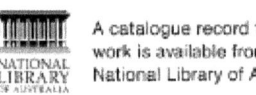 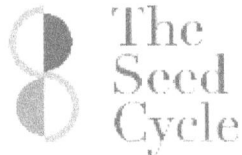

Disclaimer: The information presented in this book authored by Melissa Kovacevic CEO of The Seed Cycle™ Company is intended for educational purposes only. It is not intended to be a substitute for professional medical advice, diagnosis, or treatment. Always seek the advice of your physician or another qualified healthcare provider with any questions you may have regarding a medical condition. Never disregard professional medical advice or delay in seeking it because of something you have read in this book. If you have a medical condition or are taking medications, consult with your healthcare provider before making any changes to your diet or lifestyle. Melissa Kovacevic and The Seed Cycle™ Company do not provide medical advice or treatment recommendations. For more information about the author visit www.theseedcycle.au.

Dedication

Isabella, Sebastian, and the Sisterhood.

For my children and the remarkable women whose unwavering support and inspiration light my path.

I acknowledge the Ngunnawal people, the Traditional Custodians of the land on which this book was written, and pay my respects to their Elders past, present, and emerging. I also recognise the rich and continuing traditions of Indigenous cultures, particularly their knowledge of food as medicine, which continues to inspire and educate us today.

In this book, while I primarily refer to women and females in discussions surrounding menstruation and hormonal health, I acknowledge and honour the diversity of individuals who experience menstruation. I recognise that not all individuals who menstruate identify as women, which is why The Seed Cycle™, as company and community strives to create a welcoming and inclusive space for everyone, regardless of gender identity or expression. My goal is to provide valuable insights and support for all individuals navigating the complexities of menstrual health and wellness, ensuring that everyone feels seen, respected, and empowered on their unique journey.

Contents

Foreword by Cyndi O'Meara 1
The meaning behind Seeds of Sisterhood 5
Introduction 7
Chapter 1 Medicine Women, Food and Mother Nature 9
Chapter 2 Functional Nutrition, EFT and Our Body's Innate Intelligence 19
Chapter 3 Endocrine System: Hormone Imbalances 33
Chapter 4 Sisterhood, The Red Tent and the Moon 49
Chapter 5 Cyclical Rhythms and The Menstrual Cycle 59
Chapter 6 Origins of Seed Cycling 75
Chapter 7 Seed Cycling Nutrients, Science and Research 87
Chapter 8 Seed Cycling Benefits and How to Get Started 113
Chapter 9 Seed Cycling for PMS, the Pill and Teens 131
Chapter 10 Menopause and Seed Cycling 145
Chapter 11 Seed Cycling for PCOS and Other Conditions ... 155
Chapter 12 Seed Cycling Recipes 163
    Hormone Helper Seed Cycle Snaps 166
    Seed Cycle + Protein Smoothie Recipes 168
    Seed Cycle Harmony Bliss Balls 169
    Seed + Oat Salmon Nourish Bowl Recipe 170
    Phase 1 Vegan Seed Cycle Brownie Bites Recipe 172
    Seed Cycling Phase 2 Chocolate Raspberry Bars 174
    Seed Cycle Crackers Recipe 176
    Choc Rice Puffs Recipe 178
    Seed Cycle Yoghurt Bowl Recipe 180
    Goodbye PMS Avocado Choc Mousse Recipe 182

    Estrogen Detox Carrot & Lentil Salad Recipe 184

    Hormone Support Green Banana Flour Pancakes 186

    Seed Cycle Toast Toppers 188

    Seed Cycling 189

Acknowledgments 191

The Seed Cycle™ Resources 192

Recommendations: Books and Courses 193

References 195

Index 232

Foreword by Cyndi O'Meara

When you study the endocrine (hormone) system, you realise the complexity of all the organs, hormones, regulators, negative and positive feedback loops and all the other things we still have not discovered. Both males and females are complex, but the female trumps the complexity.

Our hormones and cycles are dictated by every aspect of our lives. Including but not limited to, movement, food, sunshine, moon cycles, circadian health, sleep, family matters (pregnant, breast feeding or not), stress (perceived and imagined) grounding, health, inflammatory processes and so much more. If you do not embrace all for your health, you may miss an important puzzle piece in your health and fertility journey.

I feel that modern medicine has made the female body and its hormones and cycles and menopause and now perimenopause a disease, to be managed with medications. But when you see the complexity of the endocrine system you see that it's not that easy. It is not black and white, it's very multi-faceted. And when you throw a medication in the mix, is messes with the whole system, not just the skin, cycle and or pain but every part of your hormone system and body health.

I believe as is the philosophy of Vitalism, that the human body is an innate intelligence that is more complex than science and medicine has figured out. How have we survived and been fertile, without disease and without modern medicine? It's simple. We lived by the laws of nature and evolved with nature and all it has to offer. It is only now that the science is catching up and understands the complexity of health and that it cannot be found in a pill.

My first year of university I studied Anthropology and Cultural Anthropology, it was an awakening for me. I realised that we evolved to live in an environment with specific foods, depending on that environment, along with the cycles of the sun, moon and stars along with living in the elements of hot and cold and having an active outdoor life grounding on the earth, bathing in the waters and walking through the forests or deserts.

The comforts of modern life and the convenience of ultra processed foods and medications has changed all that. We live in airconditioned houses, drive airconditioned cars, we've lost touch with the sun and the moon, we don't go barefoot as we should, we have no extremes in temperature, we don't have time to prepare real food, we live in a chemical soup including agriculture, personal care products, food and medications, our sleep patterns are disturbed by bright lights and as a result men have a declining sperm count and women's fertility is decreasing at an unprecedented rate.

Not only that but thyroid disease (one of the parts of the endocrine system) is rising, stress and the term 'adrenal fatigue' is becoming a household name, our master hormone leptin is not being listened to by the body due to the increase in obesity and many of the other parts of the endocrine system as well as all their messengers do not have the right ingredients to do their job correctly.

Now I'm not saying you must give up modern life, but what you must do is fake it so that your evolutionary body believes it is still living as a hunter gatherer.

Allopathic medicine (meaning all passive) has a diagnosis and medication ready for you. But if you are prepared to not be 'all passive' and change what you eat, how you live, your lifestyle then I've seen miracles happen.

Melissa Kovacevic has put together the Seeds of Sisterhood. It made me proud to be a woman, her ancient wisdom that she has collated gave me a sense of history in who I am and how powerful the female body is at every stage of our lives.

I'm on the other side of menopause. I was fortunate to be bought up in a family that believed in the great outdoors of camping and picnics. My family also had the belief that the human body is an innate intelligence, feed it the right foods, give it the right ingredients for health and it can be the healthiest it can possibly be. I'm 64. I do not and have not taken any medications. I've breezed through every aspect of my cycles. I hiked and camped in the wilds for 60 days through the Colorado

Rockies, Utah National Parks and Grand Canyon without bother of pain or my cycle when I was 20.

The pill in my family was seen as poison and my mother taught me the power of my cycle and how to read it for fertility and non-fertility. I became pregnant when I planned, had wonderfully easy births and my last was at home, I breast feed without issue and I didn't lose a day to sickness because of my cycle, I realised that menopause had happened without fanfare and now at 64 I ocean swim, barefoot sand run and bike every day before 7.30am just so my body thinks it lives in nature and the wilds and so I see the sunrise and create incredible circadian health. I'm addicted to my morning routine. I live in a modern home, but I make sure my body thinks it lives in the wilds. I consume only real foods as I know that it nourishes my body, and it is the only food that is recognised by my evolutionary body.

Most doctors call me lucky, but I call it good management. The sad thing is that most parents and most people have been hoodwinked into a very different paradigm for health, all passive is the catch cry. You can break that cycle, so that things change.

Seeds of Sisterhood makes you proud to be a woman, it gives you the tools to change what you are going through. It is no good reading this book and doing nothing, you must become responsible for your health by taking action with your foods, using seed cycling, managing stress, changing paradigms and becoming educated.

There is a change happening, people are waking up. I was lucky my parents were awake in the 1950's. I believe this book can wake more people up so that they do not suffer the consequences of the masses. If you continue to do what everyone else is doing you will continue to get the same result. If you continue to do what you are doing you will continue to get the same result. In order to get something different you must change, and I can guarantee you a different result.

Follow the guidance of a woman (the author) who has been through this and found her way out of the maze into a world of health, love, caring, education, leadership and awakening. She was not bought up like me she had health issues, but she educated herself, took responsibility and walked out of the fog.

Her lessons are lifechanging. Her book is warming, comforting, embracing and educational. As I read her book, I felt like I was blanketed in hope and I know this sounds odd, but like I was being embraced by every woman who had walked this earth.

Thank you, Melissa Kovacevic, for being a student once and now an incredible educator. We need more women like you.

Cyndi O'Meara - Nutritionist, Author, Speaker, Founder of Changing Habits, Changing Habits Farm, The Nutrition Academy and co-founder of The Packing Company. Creator of The Changing Habits Retreats, Festival of Food and Farming, as well as the annual Health and Nutrition Summit.

The meaning behind Seeds of Sisterhood

"Seeds"

Seeds are nutritional powerhouses, providing a rich array of vitamins, minerals, and healthy fats essential for human health.

In their simplicity and abundance, seeds are a testament to nature's ability to provide us with the fundamental building blocks of health and vitality.

Metaphorically, seeds are the embodiment of potential, growth, and nourishment. They hold the promise of new beginnings, encapsulating the essence of life in their tiny forms.

"Sisterhood"

Sisterhood has been celebrated in various ways throughout history and culture. It's not just about familial ties but a symbol of strength, solidarity, and empowerment. The concept of "sisterhood" was pivotal during the women's liberation movement of the 1960s and 1970s, emphasising unity and collective action among women.

To encapsulate, sisterhood is an ancient, powerful, female force that connects women across time and space, providing a sense of belonging and unwavering support.

"Seeds of Sisterhood"

Seeds of Sisterhood intertwines the feminine spirit with the natural world, highlighting how both the nurturing energy of women and the vitality within seeds contribute to growth and strength. In this book, seeds symbolise more than their botanical essence; they represent the immense potential within every woman. Just as seeds require care, the right conditions, and time to flourish, so do women need support, love, and the understanding of their sisterhood to truly thrive.

To me, 'The Sisterhood' embodies the women who have shaped my life—extending beyond family to include friends, colleagues, teachers and women within my wider network. It represents a deep, unspoken bond that transcends mere words. This connection is ancient and powerful, inherent in our very being, binding us together through shared experiences and a shared feminine energy.

Introduction

As I sit down to share my story with you, I can't help but reflect on the journey that led me here. My name is Melissa (Mel) Kovacevic, and like many women, my relationship with food and my body has been tumultuous, shaped by the relentless pressures of diet culture and the incessant desire to fit into society's standards of beauty.

During my teens and twenties, I was trapped in a vicious cycle of diets, always chasing after the ideal of being thin. No matter how hard I tried, the numbers on the scale never matched what I wanted. Instead, my body rebelled. I had skin breakouts, and my digestion was a mess, leading to chronic constipation. Mentally, I was in a dark place, constantly feeling depressed and anxious.

Looking back, I realise now that this cycle of dieting was not just about losing weight—it was about seeking validation, acceptance, and control in a world that often made me feel inadequate. It's a cycle that many of us find ourselves trapped in, as we succumb to the promises of quick fixes and fad diets, only to find ourselves back at square one, feeling more disheartened than ever.

But through it all, there was a small seed of hope planted within me—a seed that would eventually blossom into a revolutionary approach to women's health and wellness.

Growing up in a Croatian household, food wasn't just sustenance—it was and still is a cornerstone of our culture, a source of comfort and connection. I have fond memories of my grandparents' vegetable garden, bursting with vibrant colours and fragrant herbs. And oh, the cakes my grandma would bake, rich with butter, milled nuts, and decadent chocolate! Homemade bread, pasta, and hearty soups were staples of our kitchen, lovingly prepared and shared around the family table. But as I fell deeper into the grip of diet culture, I began to distance myself from these cherished traditions. I turned away from the foods that had once brought me so much joy, fearing them. Family gatherings became a source of anxiety, as I struggled to resist the temptation of dishes laden with what I deemed to be "too much fat." How wrong I was!

One day, fed up with the endless cycle of restrictive diets and futile weight loss efforts, I hit rock bottom. Fresh off an exhausting 8-week gym challenge with its narrow list of approved foods, I found myself trapped in a vicious cycle of binge eating and self-loathing. It was then that a thought occurred to me: what if I studied nutrition? Perhaps then, I could finally unlock the secret to weight loss.

My journey into the world of nutrition began with basic studies, where I learned the fundamentals of food and its impact on the body. But it wasn't until I delved into the realm of Functional Nutrition that my perspective underwent a profound transformation. Here, I discovered the concept of food as medicine—a powerful tool for healing and nourishing the body from within. Guided by the principles of vitalism and armed with the latest breakthroughs in epigenetics and gut health, I began to see health in a whole new light.

Yet, despite my newfound knowledge and understanding, I found myself grappling with deep-rooted self-limiting beliefs and negative patterns of behaviour. It was then that I turned to Emotional Freedom Techniques (EFT) or Tapping, a powerful tool for releasing emotional blockages and restoring balance to the mind and body. Through the practice of EFT, I began to unravel the tangled web of fears and insecurities that had long held me captive, allowing me to reclaim control of my life and my health.

But even as EFT brought me closer to wholeness, there remained a missing piece of the puzzle. It wasn't until I began listening to the stories of women that I stumbled upon a common thread—a shared struggle that resonated with each one of them.

And it is this revelation, this shared experience, that holds the key to unlocking the next chapter in my journey—and theirs.

Chapter 1
Medicine Women, Food and Mother Nature

With deep gratitude and profound respect, I honour the remarkable women throughout history who have paved the way for harnessing the healing potential of food. These revered figures, known as medicine women or healers, have left a lasting mark by embracing natural remedies and holistic healing practices.

Did you know that historically, healing was often seen as a natural and nurturing role embraced by women, mothers and wives? Women played crucial roles in their communities, offering healing and wisdom through their knowledge of herbal remedies, dietary practices, and intuitive wisdom.

Healing has been an inherent responsibility passed down from mother to daughter, friend to friend, and generation to generation. It was—and remains—a sacred act of sisterhood, a shared wisdom where one woman's strength becomes the strength of many.

From ancient Greece to medieval Europe, from indigenous tribes to modern-day practitioners, women have left an indelible mark on the history of medicine and continue to inspire us with their insights into the healing power of food.

Through their wisdom and compassion, these women have not only healed bodies but also empowered others to take charge of their health and reclaim their connection to nature. Their legacies remind us of the profound relationship between food and medicine, and the importance of honouring and preserving traditional healing practices.

The Lost Knowledge of Medicine Women

Throughout history, there have been instances where the knowledge, wisdom, and writings of medicine women, herbalists, and healers were suppressed, destroyed, or intentionally hidden. This suppression occurred because of various factors, including patriarchal structures, religious persecution, and political agendas.

Here are a few examples:

> **Witch Hunts and Persecution:** During the witch hunts of the Middle Ages and Early Modern period, thousands of women accused of witchcraft were subjected to torture, trials, and execution. Many of these women were healers, midwives, or herbalists who held knowledge of medicinal plants and natural remedies. Their practices were often seen as a threat to established medical authorities and religious institutions, leading to their persecution and the destruction of their writings and teachings.
>
> **Colonialism and Cultural Suppression:** In colonised regions around the world, indigenous healing traditions and knowledge were often denigrated or suppressed by colonial powers. European colonisers imposed their own medical systems and dismissed the healing practices of indigenous peoples as primitive or superstitious. As a result, valuable insights into traditional herbal medicine and food-based healing practices were marginalised or lost.
>
> **Medicalisation of Healthcare:** With the rise of modern medicine and the dominance of pharmaceuticals in healthcare, traditional healing practices and herbal remedies were often relegated to the margins of society. It is said that medical authorities and regulatory bodies sought to standardise medical treatments and suppress alternative therapies deemed

unscientific or unconventional. This led to the marginalisation and censorship of traditional healers and their knowledge.

Library and Manuscript Destruction: Throughout history, libraries and repositories of knowledge were targeted for destruction during times of conflict, war or conquest. One example of this is the Library of Ashurbanipal in ancient Assyria destroyed when Nineveh was sacked by invading armies in the 7th century BCE. Ancient texts, manuscripts, and scrolls containing valuable information about herbal medicine and healing practices were lost or destroyed, depriving future generations of invaluable wisdom and insights.

Despite these challenges, fragments of ancient wisdom and knowledge have survived through oral traditions, hidden manuscripts, and obscure texts. In recent years, there has been a resurgence of interest in traditional healing practices, leading to efforts to preserve and revive indigenous knowledge and reclaim ancestral healing traditions. By honouring the legacy of medicine women and rediscovering their teachings, we can reclaim lost wisdom and reconnect with the healing power of food and nature.

The Story of Agnodice

Join me as I share the story of Agnodice to pay tribute to the medicine women who have paved the way for the use of food as medicine, celebrating their enduring legacy and the timeless wisdom they have bestowed upon us.

The story of Agnodice resonates deeply with me due to my personal connection to women's health through my maternal lineage. From an early age, I witnessed the challenges and strength surrounding reproductive health in my family. This experience shaped my understanding of the vital role women play in supporting one another. Agnodice's story embodies the courage to break barriers and care for others—something that aligns with my own journey.

In ancient Greece, during a time when women were often marginalised and barred from practicing medicine, there lived a legendary figure named Agnodice. Though her existence is shrouded in the mists of time, her story echoes through the ages, symbolising the resilience of women in the field of medicine.

Agnodice dared to defy the conventions of her era, breaking free from the constraints that confined women to the domestic sphere. Disguising herself as a man, she boldly stepped into the realm of medicine, where few women had dared to tread before.

With boundless courage and unwavering determination, Agnodice pursued her calling as a healer, specialising in the delicate art of obstetrics and gynaecology. In a society where women's health concerns were often overlooked or dismissed, Agnodice became a beacon of hope for countless women in need of care and compassion.

Through her skilled hands and compassionate heart, Agnodice brought comfort and solace to women during the sacred moments of childbirth, guiding them through the trials and triumphs of motherhood. She listened to their fears and whispered words of encouragement, offering not only medical expertise but also a nurturing presence that eased their anxieties.

Despite the challenges and obstacles, she faced, Agnodice remained undaunted in her mission to serve her fellow women. Her dedication and devotion earned her the admiration and respect of all who knew her, and her name became synonymous with courage and compassion in the field of medicine.

Though the historical accuracy of Agnodice's existence may be debated, her legacy endures as a powerful symbol of women's contributions to the healing arts. Agnodice stands as a testament to the strength and resilience of women throughout history, inspiring future generations to pursue their passions and break barriers in the pursuit of knowledge and healing.

Food as Medicine

In our modern world, where quick fixes and pharmaceuticals often dominate the healthcare landscape, the concept of food as medicine stands as a powerful testament to the healing potential of nature's bounty. Rooted in centuries-old wisdom, at its core, food as medicine is a practice grounded in the understanding that the foods we eat play a crucial role in disease prevention and management.

The Origins of Food as Medicine

Food as medicine has ancient origins and can be traced back to various cultures throughout history. Some of the earliest documented texts on the use of food for therapeutic purposes originate from ancient civilisations such as China, India, and Greece.

In China, the practice of using food as medicine is deeply rooted in traditional Chinese medicine (TCM), which dates back thousands of years. The Huangdi Neijing, or Yellow Emperor's Inner Canon, is one of the oldest and most influential texts in TCM. It emphasises the importance of diet and nutrition in maintaining health and preventing disease, outlining principles for selecting foods based on their energetic properties and therapeutic effects on the body.

Similarly, in India, the ancient Ayurvedic texts provide detailed guidance on dietary practices for promoting health and treating various ailments. The Charaka Samhita and Sushruta Samhita, among other Ayurvedic texts, describe the medicinal properties of different foods and spices and prescribe specific dietary regimens tailored to individual constitutions (doshas) and health conditions.

For Indigenous Australians, the use of food as medicine is deeply ingrained in cultural traditions that span thousands of years. Traditional Aboriginal and Torres Strait Islander healing practices are centred around a holistic understanding of health, incorporating the physical, spiritual, and environmental dimensions of well-being. The rich biodiversity of Australia's landscapes provided Indigenous communities with an abundance of medicinal plants, bush foods, and natural resources, which were utilised for their healing properties.

From the nutritious fruits of native bush tucker such as Kakadu plum and quandong to the medicinal qualities of plants like tea tree, eucalyptus, and kangaroo apple, Indigenous Australians developed a sophisticated understanding of the therapeutic benefits of local flora. Healing ceremonies, known as "corroborees" or "cleansing ceremonies," often included the consumption of specific foods and the application of natural remedies to promote health and vitality. Despite the disruptions and dislocations caused by colonisation, many Indigenous communities continue to uphold and revitalise traditional healing practices, recognising the enduring wisdom of their ancestors and the importance of food as medicine in maintaining cultural resilience and connection to country.

A Root Cause Approach

A root cause approach or Root Cause Analysis (RCA) emphasises identifying and addressing the fundamental underlying factors that contribute to a person's overall well-being, rather than simply treating symptoms of illness. This holistic methodology seeks to understand the complex interplay of lifestyle, genetic, environmental, and psychosocial factors that impact health.

Integrating a root cause approach into modern healthcare aligns with ancient principles and effectively addresses the limitations of a symptom-focused model. This approach recognises that true healing involves identifying and treating the underlying causes of health issues, rather than merely managing symptoms.

I do wonder why RCA is not more widely adopted in Western medicine? Is it because current practices often emphasise immediate symptom relief over exploring deeper causes?

I envision a future where RCA is embraced globally, driving more sustainable and preventive healthcare practices. Personally, I apply this approach for myself and my family. This mindset helps us address underlying issues rather than just managing surface-level symptoms.

Functional Foods

One of the key pillars of food as medicine are functional foods—foods that not only provide sustenance but also offer physiological benefits beyond basic nutrition.

Functional foods are rich sources of micronutrients, antioxidants, and bioactive compounds that have been shown to support optimal health and reduce the risk of chronic diseases. From vibrant herbs and spices to humble legumes, nuts, and seeds, functional foods encompass a diverse array of natural wonders that can nourish and heal the body from within.

Functional foods can be referred to by several alternate names, including medicinal foods, nutritional foods, nutraceuticals, prescriptive foods, therapeutic foods, superfoods, and foodceuticals. Let's explore the differences between these definitions, as there are subtle distinctions among them. I anticipate that clearer definitions and categories will emerge in the future.

Nutraceuticals

Nutraceuticals, a fusion of "nutrition" and "pharmaceuticals," represent a flourishing field at the intersection of food and medicine. From herbal extracts and vitamins to probiotics and Omega-3 fatty acids, nutraceuticals aim to promote overall health as well as prevent disease, and even treat certain health conditions. As we are increasingly seeking natural alternatives to conventional medicine, nutraceuticals have gained popularity for their potential to support various aspects of health, including immune function, cognitive health, and cardiovascular wellness.

However, as with any category, there exists a spectrum ranging from outstanding products to heavily manufactured foods and supplements labelled as healthy. When selecting a product or supplement, I pose the question, "Does this originate from nature?" and inquire about the manufacturing and production processes involved in creating the product.

I have recently become more interested in who owns the companies I buy from and their ethical practices. I like to do my research because I believe in "voting with my dollar"—supporting companies that align with my values. If I am unsure, I find out who owns the company and consult with them to ensure their practices align with my standards and values.

So, what are my standards and values? For me, this involves looking for transparency in sourcing and sustainability in production. For instance, when checking the ingredients on a product, if I see additives like artificial colours or preservatives, it raises a red flag for me about the overall quality and ethics of the company. I also prioritise companies that are environmentally friendly.

Foodceuticals

I am particularly intrigued by the term "foodceutical" as I believe it offers a compelling category for The Seed Cycle™ products.

Foodceuticals, though not widely acknowledged, encapsulates a category of nature-based functional foods renowned for their intrinsic therapeutic properties and health benefits that transcend basic nutrition. These products, abundant in bioactive compounds, deliver physiological advantages in enhancing overall health and well-being. Unlike nutraceuticals, which may contain synthesised or isolated compounds, foodceuticals emphasise only natural sources.

Mother Nature

Mother Nature—also known as Mother Earth, Gaia, Demeter, or by other names in different cultures—is a deeply revered embodiment of the natural world. Across countless civilisations and mythologies, she symbolises the nurturing, life-giving, and sustaining aspects of the Earth. Through mother nature, we recognise the interconnectedness of all living beings with the environment and acknowledge the Earth as a provider of resources, fertility, and abundance.

Mother Nature is often depicted as a maternal figure, embodying qualities of compassion, wisdom, and resilience. She nurtures and sustains life through the growth of plants and forests, the flow of rivers, and the diversity of wildlife. Many traditions honour her through rituals, ceremonies, and prayers, expressing gratitude for her bountiful gifts and her role in sustaining the web of life.

Ancient Mesopotamian texts associate her with the goddess Inanna or Ishtar, symbolising the fertility of the land and agricultural cycles. In ancient Egyptian mythology, the goddess Isis represented fertility and nature, embodying nurturing and protective qualities. Similarly, in Greek mythology, Gaia personified the Earth and represented the primal mother from whom all life emerged.

As we push forward in this modern era, we often neglect the wisdom of the ages, losing respect for Mother Nature by believing we can outsmart her through science and technology.

I see companies attempting to replicate nutrients in lab-made foods and supplements, moving us further away from real, whole foods. Beyond that, modern agriculture is driven by synthetic fertilisers, pesticides, and genetically modified crops, aiming to increase yield but often depleting the soil's natural nutrients and biodiversity. Livestock are raised with growth hormones and antibiotics, disconnecting us from the natural cycles of food production. Even in our pursuit of convenience and efficiency, we've overlooked the inherent wisdom of nature's balance, believing that we can recreate what she has perfected over millennia. These artificial shortcuts may offer temporary solutions but ultimately leave us with food systems that are less nutritious, less sustainable, and less in harmony with the Earth.

Yet, I hope we come to realise that we can never surpass the brilliance of nature itself. True wisdom lies in respecting Mother Earth and working in harmony with her natural systems. By embracing this approach, we can harness the healing power of real food, promote lasting health, and maintain a sustainable relationship with nature—for ourselves and for future generations.

In the chapters that follow, we will delve deeper into the specific ways in which food as medicine can support hormonal health— A journey that begins with understanding our unique and incredible endocrine system, and the role of nutrient-rich foods, among much more, in achieving hormonal balance.

Chapter 2
Functional Nutrition, EFT and Our Body's Innate Intelligence

Following the birth of my daughter, I was filled with a newfound sense of determination and self-confidence, a transformation that can follow a challenging, life-altering experience. I vividly recall thinking, "If I can birth and breastfeed a baby, there's nothing I can't do!"

During my maternity leave, I experienced a profound shift in my life. For the first time as an adult, I had the luxury of space — both physically and emotionally. This newfound freedom allowed me to step outside, bask in the beauty of nature, and embrace moments of pure connection with my baby, family, friends, and even strangers. I noticed I was enjoying new conversations with people I met out and about, something that hadn't happened often in the past. Lots of people chat with you when you have a cute baby with you!

I felt liberated, inspired, and deeply connected to myself in a way I had never experienced before. It was a time of unparalleled growth and self-discovery, as I navigated the journey of motherhood with a sense of freedom and wonder.

I recognise that my journey may not reflect the experiences of all mothers, and I deeply appreciate the privilege of having space from workforce pressures, as well as the physical and mental safety afforded to myself and my family during this transformative time.

I found myself in a place of harmony with food and my body, a place where I felt as though I had discovered the elusive key to self-love and acceptance. Yet, as I looked around me, I witnessed other women still ensnared in the very struggles I had once faced. They grappled with food, overexercising, obsessive calorie counting, restriction, unhealthy fixation on their bodies, and so much self-criticism.

As I reflected on my own journey of healing, a powerful realisation dawned upon me: I possessed the knowledge and tools to facilitate healing in others. It was a moment of clarity where I understood that my experiences were not just for my own benefit, but also an opportunity to extend a helping hand to those in similar struggles.

I felt a deep-seated sense of responsibility to share the transformative practices that had brought me freedom. It became clear to me that I had the capacity to make a meaningful difference in the lives of others, offering them a pathway towards healing, resilience, and health. I made the decision to embark on the journey of entrepreneurship, completing my practitioner accreditations and founding my own business to offer Functional Nutrition and Clinical Emotional Freedom Techniques (EFT) sessions.

My mission was clear: to create a safe, supportive space where individuals could embark on their journey of healing and self-discovery, no longer facing their challenges alone.

With deep gratitude for the wisdom and guidance of my teachers and mentors, I established my practice to assist others, peer to peer, in reconnecting with their bodies and tapping into their innate intelligence. By teaching mindful, intuitive eating and offering education on whole-food nutrition, alongside the transformative practice of EFT, I set out to empower people to reclaim ownership of their health.

Introduction to Functional Nutrition

Functional Nutrition is a dynamic approach to health that delves beyond the traditional focus solely on nutrients. It considers the intricate interplay between lifestyle choices, environmental factors, emotional well-being, and overall health. At its core, Functional Nutrition embraces a vitalistic philosophy, viewing the body as an integrated system where each component influences the other.

My journey into Functional Nutrition began with my Chiropractor and Kinesiologist, Fiona Glenn, who introduced me to the renowned Australian nutritionist Cyndi O'Meara. Cyndi is celebrated for her pioneering work in Functional Nutrition, empowering individuals to take charge of their health through education and whole food-based nutrition. She has devoted her life to challenging conventional beliefs and fostering a holistic and vitalistic understanding of health. I am incredibly grateful to have had the opportunity to learn from her.

Understanding Functional Nutrition

Functional Nutrition approaches health from a holistic perspective, recognising that optimal well-being is achieved through a comprehensive understanding of the body's interconnected systems. Instead of focusing solely on treating symptoms,

Functional Nutrition aims to address the root causes of health challenges and nutritional issues. At its core, this approach emphasizes the importance of personalised, food-based recommendations tailored to individual needs. Rather than relying exclusively on isolated nutrients or supplements, Functional Nutrition encourages the consumption of whole, nutrient-dense foods that support the body's natural processes.

Integral to the philosophy of Functional Nutrition is the principle of vitalism. Vitalism acknowledges that our bodies possess an innate intelligence, capable of adaptation, healing, and thriving when provided with the right tools and resources. This philosophy transforms the way we perceive our bodies, shifting our focus inward to listen to the cues and signals they provide.

For many, including myself, embracing the vitalistic philosophy of Functional Nutrition has been transformative. It has empowered me to turn inward for information about my body, learning to interpret the subtle cues that indicate my nutritional needs. Instead of relying solely on external sources for guidance, I have come to recognise the wisdom inherent within my own body.

For instance, I've learned to listen to my hunger cues, understanding that cravings for certain foods, like leafy greens or healthy fats, often signal a need for specific nutrients. Additionally, I pay attention to how my body feels after meals—if I feel sluggish after a meal, it reinforces my desire to prioritise whole, nutrient-dense options.

Many people ask me about the difference between Functional Medicine and Functional Nutrition, and here's my perspective: Functional Medicine is a holistic approach addressing the root causes of disease, while Functional Nutrition focuses specifically on the role of nutrition in supporting healing and health.

Historical Perspectives on Nutrition

A fundamental aspect of Functional Nutrition involves examining nutrition through a historical lens, drawing insights from the diets of our ancestors. By studying the eating habits of ancient cultures and traditional societies, we gain valuable insights into the dietary patterns that sustained human health for millennia.

Our ancestors had a deep connection to their food sources, consuming a diverse array of nutrient-rich foods obtained through hunting, gathering, and local farming. Their diets were rich in whole, minimally processed foods, providing a balanced array of essential nutrients to support overall health.

In contrast to modern diets characterised by processed foods, refined sugars, and synthetic additives, traditional diets were inherently nutrient-dense and aligned with the body's natural needs. By embracing ancestral nutrition, Functional Nutrition reconnects us with past wisdom to promote optimal health.

Today, this might look like:

- Sourcing locally produced foods for freshness and nutrient density.
- Making meals from scratch instead of relying on processed substitutes.
- Meal prepping on weekends to save time during the week.
- Using simple, quick recipes that prioritise whole ingredients.
- Involving the family in cooking to make it enjoyable and efficient.

These practices help integrate ancestral wisdom into our busy lives. In doing so, we cultivate a lifestyle that honours the health-sustaining practices of our ancestors while adapting them to meet the demands of modern living, and we can create a harmonious balance between tradition and convenience.

Mindful and Intuitive Eating Practices

Another key aspect of Functional Nutrition involves shifting away from the popular calorie-in, calorie-out, macros and deficit approach to nutrition, and instead, embracing mindful and intuitive eating practices.

Research indicates that those who practice intuitive eating are less likely to engage in disordered eating behaviours and are more likely to appreciate their bodies. Studies have shown that intuitive eating is associated with lower body mass index (BMI), better psychological health, and a more positive body image compared to those who follow restrictive dieting patterns.

I can attest to the transformative power of these practices. Mindful and intuitive eating helped me improve my relationship with food as well as manage my weight, this approach is not a one-time fix but an ongoing practice and focus that continues to bring me food and body freedom. Mindful eating, stemming from the Buddhist concept of mindfulness, emphasises being fully present during meals.

> *Have you practiced focusing on the taste, texture, and aroma of your food?*
>
> *How does this mindful approach affect your eating experience and satisfaction?*

Intuitive eating, on the other hand, encourages trusting your body's signals and eating without judgment, focusing on nourishment rather than restriction. How do you distinguish between physical hunger and emotional cravings? To practice mindful and intuitive eating, start by eliminating distractions during meals, such as turning off the TV or putting away your phone.

Take time to appreciate the colours, textures, and flavours of your food. Eat slowly, chew thoroughly, and listen to your body's signals of hunger and fullness. Reflect on how different foods make you feel, both physically and emotionally.

The benefits of these practices are profound. By cultivating a mindful approach to eating, you are more likely to develop a healthier relationship with food, reducing instances of overeating or emotional eating. This can lead to better weight management, improved digestion, and increased satisfaction with your meals.

You Are What You Eat

The saying "You are what you eat" is a powerful reminder of how our food choices impact our overall health, especially our skin. I once heard a concept that has always stayed with me and guides my food choices. "Imagine your skin as a reflection of your diet." If you are consuming ultra-processed foods or, for instance, live off rice crackers (as I once did), your skin will likely be dry and lifeless, mirroring the lack of nutrients in your diet. However, if you nourish your body with beautiful, colourful foods like seeds, ghee, dahl, soups, and broths, your skin will be hydrated, vibrant, and full of life. Eating nutrient-dense foods rich in vitamins, minerals, and antioxidants not only supports my overall health but also gives my skin a radiant, healthy glow.

Introduction to EFT Tapping

Emotional Freedom Techniques (EFT) also known as Tapping is a powerful and versatile tool for promoting emotional well-being and reducing stress. Developed in the 1990s by Gary Craig, EFT combines elements of Eastern acupressure with modern psychology to address emotional issues and physical discomfort. At its core, EFT is based on the premise that unresolved emotional issues can contribute to physical symptoms and health imbalances.

EFT involves gently tapping on specific meridian points on the body while focusing on emotional triggers or distressing thoughts. This tapping sequence is accompanied by verbal affirmations or statements that acknowledge the issue being addressed. By stimulating these meridian points while tuning into the emotion, EFT aims to release energetic blockages and restore balance to the body's energy system.

The Science Behind EFT Tapping

Research shows that EFT helps to regulate the body's stress response and reduce levels of cortisol, the stress hormone. Studies have also shown that EFT can lead to improvements in psychological symptoms such as anxiety, depression, and post-traumatic stress disorder (PTSD). Additionally, brain imaging studies have demonstrated changes in brain activity following EFT sessions, indicating its potential impact on the brain's emotional processing centres.

Practical Applications of EFT Tapping

EFT can be employed to address a wide range of emotional challenges, from everyday stress and anxiety to more complex issues like trauma and phobias. It can also be integrated into various holistic wellness practices, including Functional Nutrition and meditation, to support overall health and well-being.

For me, EFT was instrumental in helping me uncover and release the underlying core beliefs behind my food issues and obsession with being thin. I held the belief that I needed to be skinny to be loved. During times of anxiety and self-doubt, I practiced EFT while looking in the mirror, allowing myself to confront and express my feelings. Additionally, I worked with EFT practitioners who guided me in releasing these old beliefs, patterns, and behaviours.

My journey was significantly supported by Naomi Janzen, an Evidence-Based (EBEFT) Accredited Advanced Practitioner Trainer, who helped me navigate my own blocks and trained me to become the experienced practitioner I am today.

EFT with a Certified Practitioner

There are different forms of EFT, and it is increasingly being included as a module in broader online coaching courses. I value Evidence-Based EFT, and this is what I would recommend when looking for a practitioner. I would also always check that they are trauma-informed and trained. If you want to look for an EFT practitioner, consider those trained by EFT Universe or Peta Stapleton's Evidence-Based EFT program, or a professional institute dedicated to using Clinical EFT.

When to work with an EFT Practitioner:

- Trauma recovery
- Binge and emotional eating
- Stress and anxiety
- Depression
- Relationship issues
- EFT for kids
- Pain management
- Hormone Imbalances and menopause symptoms
- Chronic conditions

Using EFT Tapping in Daily Life

One of the greatest strengths of EFT is its accessibility and ease of use. It can be practiced virtually anywhere and at any time, making it a valuable tool for managing stress and promoting emotional resilience in daily life. Use EFT when you:

- Feel overwhelmed
- During times of stress
- After a challenging conversation
- When feeling frustrated or after an argument
- When feeling activated or triggered by an event
- When feeling guilty or after overeating
- For managing food cravings

How to do basic EFT

The process of EFT encompasses tapping the following meridian points in the following order:

- Side of the Hand (Karate Chop): Tap the fleshy, narrow side of the hand, below the little finger.
- Eyebrow Point (EB): Where the eyebrows begin, closest to the bridge of the nose.
- Side of Eye (SE): on the bone directly along the outside of either eye (also known as your temple).
- Under Eye (UE): On the bone directly under either eye.

- Under Nose (UN): The area directly beneath the nose and above the upper lip.
- Chin Point (CP): This is the area just below your bottom lip and above the chin, right in the crease.
- Collarbone Point (CB): Starting from where your collar bones meet in the centre, go down an inch and out an inch on either side.
- Under Arm (UA): On your side, about four inches beneath the armpit.
- Top of Head (TH): Directly on the crown of your head.

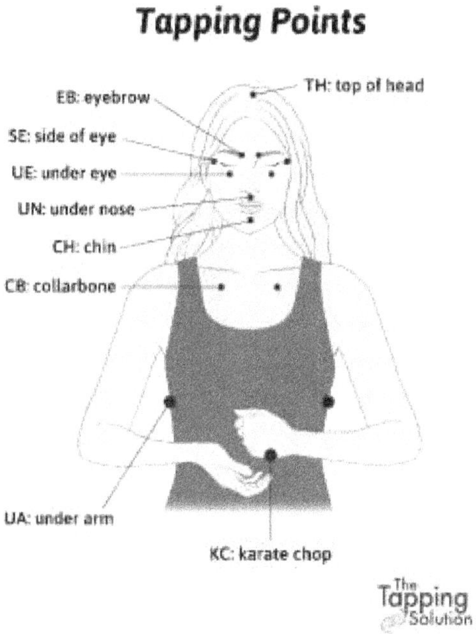

Figure 1. Tapping Points

Note. This image has been derived from The Tapping Solution, an EFT iPhone/android application

Start the EFT Sequence

STEP 1 – Focus on the problem and rate intensity. While focusing on the specific problem/negative emotion or uncomfortable physical sensation, rate on a scale from 0 to 10 (10 being maximum intensity, 0 being no intensity).

STEP 2 – Create and perform a setup phrase. While tapping on the Side of the Hand repeat your setup phrase three times: "Even though I have (this problem, uncomfortable emotion or physical sensation), I deeply and completely accept myself."

For example: "Even though I feel frustrated and hormonal, I deeply and completely accept myself."

STEP 3 – Tap through the remaining points. Start with the Top of Head and finish with the Under Arm point, tap approximately 7-10 times through each point using a reminder phrase to help you keep your attention on the energy of the problem.

For example: "The frustration because of my hormones"

STEP 4 - Reassess your intensity, refocus and repeat. Has your rating changed? What number would you give the intensity now? If your score is still higher than a 2/10, do the process again. For your subsequent rounds adjust the wording: "Even though I still have some of this remaining (insert your problem), I deeply and completely accept myself anyway. Adjusted reminder phrase: "This remaining (insert your problem)."

For example: "This remaining frustration because of my hormones."

Beginner's EFT Tapping Checklist

Follow your intuition - As you tap you can talk about your concerns, trust your instincts. There's no need for elaborate language—just speak your truth. Let your intuition guide you on how long to tap and how many rounds to do.

Am I well hydrated? This is important to ensure energy flows along the meridians while tapping.

Secondary gains - Notice is there a downside to getting over my issue? (e.g. fear of change, loss of identity, not feeling deserving). Use the EFT sequence to help release the secondary gains.

Identify aspects - What aspects are part of the specific problem or emotion I am focusing on? (e.g. sensory, emotions, memory) Pinpoint specific events, when and how did this problem manifest in my life?

Perfection is not necessary - When you're new to EFT, remembering the sequence can be challenging. That's okay—there's no single "correct" way to tap. The technique is effective even if it's not perfect. Just do your best, keep practicing, and you will start to notice the shifts.

Do I need to seek professional assistance - Please remember, some issues should not be attempted without the guidance of a qualified EFT Practitioner. There are also times where a medical doctor is required.

What happened next

As my business expanded, I took the time to listen to the experiences of women, and I noticed a common thread in what my clients were sharing with me. They described feeling as though everything fell apart just before their periods, battling skin breakouts, intense sugar cravings, irritability, and feeling overwhelmed. During menopause, some would tell me "I feel like I am losing my mind!", while others struggled with sleep disturbances and migraines. I realised the commonality was hormones - particularly our female sex hormones.

It was during this time, armed with my belief in food as medicine, I started researching and came upon seed cycling—a natural, holistic method that harnesses the power of nutrients to restore hormonal balance. Intrigued by its potential, I delved deep into research, uncovering the science behind the practice and its profound impact on women's health.

I began teaching the seed cycling practice to my clients. I witnessed remarkable transformations unfold before my eyes.

At the heart of this practice is the concept that seeds contain essential nutrients to support hormonal balance. Seed cycling involves incorporating specific seeds—flaxseeds and pumpkin seeds in the first half of the menstrual cycle, and sesame and sunflower seeds in the second half—to help regulate hormonal fluctuations.

In my sessions, I supported my clients in understanding how to seamlessly incorporate the appropriate seed dosages into their daily routines, aligned with their menstrual cycles or the phases of the moon. I provided them with ideas and recipes for adding the seeds to smoothies, salads, soups, and yoghurt, emphasising the importance of consistency and mindfulness, as it typically takes about three cycles to experience the full benefits.

It was as if the pieces of a complex puzzle were finally falling into place, revealing a pathway to balance and vitality. Each client's journey was unique, yet there was curiosity and determination woven throughout. One client shared her experience with me, describing it as nothing short of miraculous. She expressed experiencing newfound clarity, heightened energy, and a feeling of liberation from the hormonal symptoms she had once accepted as inevitable aspects of having a period.

What struck me most was the sense of relief that radiated from my clients as they reclaimed control over their bodies and their lives. Stubborn acne that had defied conventional treatments began to clear, excess weight melted away, and mood swings gave way to a newfound sense of stability. It was clear to me that this wasn't merely a superficial fix or a temporary solution. Rather, it was a holistic approach that addressed the underlying imbalances within their bodies, supporting their hormones and nurturing their bodies.

As I reflect on these transformative experiences, I am amazed by how simple practices can have such profound effects: the power of Functional Nutrition and EFT to unlock the body's inherent ability to heal and thrive. It wasn't about masking symptoms or suppressing discomfort but rather about addressing the root causes of imbalance and restoring harmony from within. With each success story, I became increasingly convinced that this integrative approach with seed cycling being at the heart, held the key to helping women not just manage their hormonal health but truly flourish in every aspect of their lives.

The Seed Cycle™ Solution

Yet, despite these successes, I soon realised that many of my clients struggled to maintain their seed cycling routine amidst their busy lives. They would forget to buy the seeds, struggle to find certified organic, were unable to grind down the seeds themselves or run out before they had a chance to replenish them, hindering their progress and leaving them feeling overwhelmed.

It was this realisation that sparked a new vision—a vision of a convenient, accessible solution that would make seed cycling effortless for women everywhere: this is how The Seed Cycle™ was born.

The Seed Cycle™ is an organisation on a mission to revolutionise women's hormone health, one seed at a time. Everything that goes into our seed cycling products are meticulously researched and/or crafted to deliver the nutrients the body will use to thrive.

As I look back on my own journey—from struggling with my weight to finding peace and healing through nutrition and holistic wellness—I'm filled with gratitude for the path that has led me here. And I'm excited to share this journey with you, as we embark together on a quest to nurture our bodies, our spirits, and the seeds of sisterhood that bind us all together.

I should also point out a part of my story that I forget to share because honestly, it's a non-issue now but worth mentioning for those who are thinking, "this is all well and good, but I desperately want to lose weight, clear my skin, stop the symptoms and feel better ASAP!" After implementing Functional Nutrition, mindful and intuitive eating principles, using EFT and the final puzzle piece for me - seed cycling, I lost 15kg and have been able to maintain this weight for over a decade. But more than that, my skin, gut health, and vitality is better than ever. I rarely get sick; I am strong, healthy, and feel vibrant.

Chapter 3
Endocrine System: Hormone Imbalances

Understanding our key female sex hormones—estrogen, progesterone, as well as testosterone is vital knowledge that many of us weren't taught but should know about our bodies.

How much do you know about their impact on your health?

These hormones orchestrate your physiological processes and influence your mood, metabolism, and more. Have you ever thought about navigating their fluctuations with understanding and mindfulness? By learning about these hormones, we can gain a newfound understanding of our health and take control in ways we never imagined possible.

Firstly, there are critical issues that are deeply concerning and impact a significant portion of the female population that I want to bring to your attention:

- Globally, 90% of women will experience at least one symptom of pre-menstrual syndrome (PMS) at some point in their lives.

- Within this group, 20-40% of women experience PMS symptoms monthly, while 2-8% suffer from pre-menstrual dysphoric disorder (PMDD).

- A staggering 8-13% of women are diagnosed with polycystic ovarian syndrome (PCOS), with up to 70% of cases going undiagnosed globally.

- It is estimated that endometriosis affects approximately 10% of women worldwide during their reproductive years. On average, there is a delay of about 7-10 years between the onset of symptoms and diagnosis of endometriosis.

- While on the contrary, for men a hormone imbalance such as low testosterone levels affect around 2.1% of the male population.

Clinical experts in the field validate these findings, affirming the widespread occurrence of hormone-related issues in their female clinics. They highlight the range of symptoms reported by patients and diagnostic tools like hormone panels and bloodwork that uncover the scope of hormonal imbalances in women.

Unfortunately, period problems have been under-represented and under-reported, leading to negative connotations, shame, and taboo associated with menstruation and bleeding. This cultural stigma further compounds the challenges faced by women dealing with hormone imbalances, hindering open discussions and access to appropriate care and support. By shedding light on these statistics and societal perceptions, I hope we can start to reclaim control over our hormonal health.

Understanding the Female Endocrine System

The female endocrine system is a marvellously intricate network of glands. At its heart lie the ovaries, where estrogen and progesterone, the primary female sex hormones, are produced. These hormones not only govern the menstrual cycle and reproductive health but also exert profound influences on mood, metabolism, skin health, and bone density.

Testosterone, often linked with male physiology, also plays a role in smaller amounts from the ovaries and adrenal glands. Its balanced presence alongside estrogen and progesterone is crucial for menstrual cycle health.

Situated in the brain, the hypothalamus and pituitary gland serve as command centres, orchestrating hormone production through a delicate interplay of signals. The hypothalamus releases a gonadotropin-releasing hormone (GnRH), prompting the pituitary gland to secrete luteinizing hormone (LH) and follicle-stimulating hormone (FSH). These hormones, in turn, stimulate the ovaries to produce estrogen and progesterone, ensuring the rhythmic ebb and flow of the menstrual cycle.

Later in this chapter, we will delve deeper into the importance and roles of these key hormones and their intricate interactions within the female endocrine system.

Beyond the reproductive sphere, other glands such as the pancreas, which produces insulin, and the thyroid gland, responsible for thyroid hormones, contribute significantly to the endocrine symphony. Insulin regulates blood sugar levels, while thyroid hormones dictate metabolism, energy levels, and mood stability.

History of Hormone Imbalances for Women

The documentation and discussion of hormone imbalances in women can be traced back to ancient times, although the understanding of these imbalances was not as sophisticated as it is today. Ancient medical systems such as Traditional Chinese Medicine (TCM) and Ayurveda in India recognised the concept of hormonal imbalances and their effects on women's health.

In TCM, texts dating back thousands of years mention the concept of "yin" and "yang" energies and their influence on female physiology, including menstruation and fertility. Ayurvedic texts, which date back over 5,000 years, describe the role of hormones in regulating the menstrual cycle and reproductive health, as well as the use of herbs and lifestyle practices to restore hormonal balance.

In Western medicine, the formal study and documentation of hormone imbalances in women began to emerge during the 19th and early 20th centuries. With advancements in anatomy, physiology, and endocrinology, scientists and physicians started to unravel the complexities of the endocrine system and its role in regulating various bodily functions, including reproduction.

While hormone imbalances in women have gained some recognition in medical research and clinical practice today, treatment options remain limited and often revolve around medications like the oral contraceptive pill, or more invasive procedures including hysterectomies. Despite advances in diagnostic tools and treatments for conditions like polycystic ovary syndrome (PCOS) and endometriosis, many women still feel dissatisfied with the available solutions.

Regarding hysterectomies, data shows that around 600,000 hysterectomies are performed annually in the United States. However, studies have raised concerns about the necessity of many of these procedures. Research by the University of Michigan Health System in 2015 found that nearly one in five women who undergo a hysterectomy may not need the procedure, highlighting a significant number of potentially unnecessary surgeries.

There's a growing sentiment that these treatments merely manage symptoms rather than addressing the root cause of hormonal imbalances. Many women are choosing to move away from hormonal-based contraception and medication to seek natural solutions. As a result, there's a collective hope among women that future solutions will integrate ancient wisdom, body literacy, and modern science to offer more holistic and effective approaches to hormonal health.

Estrogen

Imagine estrogen as the radiant confident celebrity Taylor Swift or Beyonce of the hormone world. She arrives in the first half of the cycle, bringing energy, confidence, and a zest for life akin to their electrifying stage presence. Estrogen sets the scene, enhancing mood, sharpening memory, she supports the growth and repair of tissues, helps regulate the menstrual cycle, and even contributes to maintaining skin elasticity and hydration, giving you that glowing, youthful appearance.

Beyond these, estrogen also plays a crucial role in maintaining healthy cholesterol levels, bone health, promoting cardiovascular health and ensuring the proper functioning of the reproductive system. Estrogen is truly a powerhouse, orchestrating a symphony of wellness throughout the body.

There are three primary forms of estrogen, with a fourth form exclusively produced during pregnancy:

- Estrone (E1), originating from the ovaries, continues to play a crucial role in bone health even after menopause, albeit in reduced amounts. It serves as a reservoir estrogen, providing support beyond the reproductive years.

- Estradiol (E2), the primary estrogen during reproductive years, is pivotal in maintaining the female reproductive system and its functions. As women approach menopause, the production of estradiol decreases, impacting various aspects of health and well-being.

- Estriol (E3), predominantly synthesised in the placenta during pregnancy, supports foetal development and is also present in minor amounts in premenopausal women.

- Estetrol (E4), produced by the developing fetus during pregnancy, enhances the complexity of estrogen's functions by uniquely shaping the maternal hormonal environment and playing a vital role in regulating pregnancy-related physiological processes.

During perimenopause, the transition phase leading to menopause, estrogen levels fluctuate significantly, leading to various adjustments in the body. As women move into menopause, estrogen levels gradually decline and eventually stabilise at lower levels post-menopause.

Progesterone

Progesterone, in contrast, can be likened to Michelle Obama or even like a cozy fireplace. Progesterone enters later in the cycle with a calm and nurturing presence. She fosters stability, resilience, and inner strength, preparing the body for potential challenges ahead. Progesterone promotes relaxation, soothes anxiety, and encourages a sense of balance.

A cozy fireplace provides warmth, comfort, and a sense of home, reflecting progesterone's nurturing and stabilising qualities.

Produced primarily in the ovaries, progesterone helps prepare the uterine lining for implantation of a fertilised egg during the luteal phase of the menstrual cycleIf conception occurs, progesterone continues to be produced by the ovaries and later by the placenta, supporting the maintenance of the uterine lining and the development of the embryo and foetus.

Progesterone also exerts significant effects on various other systems in the body. In the brain, it acts as a neurosteroid*[1], influencing mood, cognition, and behaviour. Additionally, progesterone supports bone health by stimulating osteoblasts, the cells responsible for bone formation. It also plays a role in regulating fluid balance, enhancing renal function, and supporting cardiovascular health by promoting vascular smooth muscle relaxation.

Beyond its reproductive and physiological roles, progesterone is involved in modulating immune function, potentially reducing inflammation and enhancing immune response. During menopause, progesterone levels also decline, which requires the body to adjust to a new hormonal environment. Post-menopause, progesterone levels remain low, contributing to the overall shift in hormone dynamics.

Testosterone

And then there's testosterone, fearless and determined, the roaring lion or the Miley Cyrus of the hormone trio. Testosterone brings strength, drive, and assertiveness, it can embody a competitive spirit and resilience. It fuels libido, enhances muscle tone, and supports overall

---

[1]*Neurosteroids are steroid hormones synthesised in the brain or derived from peripheral sources like adrenal glands and ovaries, crossing the blood-brain barrier to directly influence neuronal activity, mood, cognition, and behaviour through modulation of neurotransmitter receptors and neuroplasticity.

vitality. It fuels determination and the ability to achieve goals with unwavering force.

Produced primarily in the ovaries and adrenal glands, testosterone contributes to various aspects of female health. It plays a role in maintaining bone density, muscle mass, and strength. Testosterone also influences libido and sexual arousal in women. Additionally, testosterone contributes to overall energy levels and mood regulation. While women have lower levels of testosterone compared to men, it is still a vital hormone for female well-being.

During menopause, testosterone levels, along with estrogen and progesterone, typically decline. However, the decline is usually more gradual compared to the sharp drops seen in estrogen and progesterone.

There are also other female sex hormones that play important roles in the body:

> **Follicle-stimulating hormone (FSH):** Produced by the pituitary gland, FSH stimulates the growth and maturation of follicles in the ovaries during the menstrual cycle. In menopause, FSH levels rise as the ovaries stop functioning, indicating the end of reproductive years.
>
> **Luteinizing hormone (LH):** Also secreted by the pituitary gland, LH triggers ovulation and the release of the egg from the ovary. In menopause, LH levels can fluctuate, contributing to symptoms such as hot flushes.
>
> **Prolactin:** Produced by the pituitary gland, prolactin plays a role in breast development and milk production during pregnancy and breastfeeding.
>
> **Androgens:** In addition to testosterone, other androgens like dehydroepiandrosterone (DHEA) and androstenedione are produced in small amounts by the adrenal glands and ovaries. They contribute to libido, muscle mass, and overall well-being in women.

Together, these hormones orchestrate a monthly symphony, each playing their unique role to maintain hormonal balance, support fertility, and influence overall health. Their rise and fall throughout the cycle reflect the intricate dance of womanhood, where each phase brings new insights, strengths, and challenges—guided by our hormonal celebrities, estrogen, progesterone, and testosterone.

I hope this overview has given you a deeper appreciation for our sex hormones and all that it provides. Its influence extends far beyond reproductive health, touching every aspect of our well-being. Recognising the vital role these hormones play can help us to support our bodies through all stages of life, from your first period (menarche) to the changes of perimenopause and beyond.

Defining Common Hormonal Imbalances

While some information presented here regarding medical and genetic conditions and disorders may extend beyond my professional expertise, it's important to understand how delicate hormone balance can impact overall health.

Disruptions in this balance can lead to various symptoms and health issues. Therefore, let's explore the research and define common hormonal imbalances. For further information and personalised support, please consult your healthcare professional.

> **Estrogen Dominance:** Estrogen dominance occurs when there is an excess of estrogen relative to progesterone in the body.
>
> **Progesterone Deficiency:** Progesterone is a crucial hormone involved in regulating the menstrual cycle and supporting pregnancy.
>
> **Thyroid Imbalance:** The thyroid gland produces hormones that regulate metabolism, energy levels, and body temperature. Imbalances in thyroid hormones, such as hypothyroidism (underactive thyroid) or hyperthyroidism (overactive thyroid), can arise from autoimmune conditions, iodine deficiency, or thyroid nodules.

Cortisol Imbalance: Cortisol is a hormone released by the adrenal glands in response to stress. Prolonged stress can lead to dysregulation of cortisol levels, resulting in adrenal fatigue.

Causes and Effects of Estrogen and Progesterone Imbalance

Understanding the causes and effects of estrogen dominance and progesterone deficiency is essential for addressing hormonal imbalances and restoring optimal health. Let's explore these imbalances in greater detail:

Causes of Estrogen Dominance:

Excessive Estrogen Production: Estrogen can be overproduced by the ovaries, especially in conditions such as estrogen-secreting tumours.

Environmental Factors: Exposure to xenoestrogens, which are synthetic compounds that mimic estrogen, can disrupt hormone balance. Xenoestrogens are commonly found in plastics, pesticides, and personal care products.

Impaired Estrogen Metabolism: Poor liver function or impaired detoxification pathways can hinder the body's ability to metabolise and eliminate excess estrogen, leading to estrogen dominance.

Genetics: Can influence the pathways involved in estrogen metabolism. Single Nucleotide Polymorphisms (SNPs) on genes like COMT and MTHFR can further impact hormone detoxification and methylation processes. These genetic variations may compromise your body's ability to efficiently metabolise and eliminate estrogen, potentially contributing to conditions associated with estrogen dominance.

Effects of Estrogen Dominance:

Irregular Menstrual Cycles: Estrogen dominance can disrupt the delicate interplay between estrogen and progesterone, resulting in irregular or heavy menstrual bleeding.

Breast Tenderness: Elevated estrogen levels can cause breast tissue to become tender, swollen, or painful, particularly in the days leading up to menstruation.

Weight Gain: Excess estrogen has been associated with increased fat deposition, particularly in the hips, thighs, and abdomen.

Mood Swings and Irritability: Fluctuations in estrogen levels can impact neurotransmitter activity in the brain, leading to mood swings, irritability, and emotional instability.

Increased Risk of Estrogen-Related Cancers: The CDC and the National Cancer Institute (NCI) highlight that longer exposure to high estrogen levels is linked to a higher risk of estrogen-related cancers like breast and uterine cancer.

Causes of Progesterone Deficiency:

Anovulation: Anovulatory cycles, where ovulation does not occur, can result in progesterone deficiency due to the absence of corpus luteum formation.

Stress-Induced Suppression: Chronic stress can disrupt the hypothalamic-pituitary-adrenal (HPA) axis, leading to reduced progesterone production and increased cortisol secretion.

Hormonal Disorders: Conditions such as PCOS or thyroid disorders can disrupt normal ovarian function, leading to progesterone deficiency.

Effects of Progesterone Deficiency:

Irregular Menstrual Cycles: Progesterone deficiency can result in irregular or absent menstrual periods, as well as anovulatory cycles.

Infertility: Progesterone plays a crucial role in preparing the uterine lining for implantation and supporting early pregnancy.

Progesterone deficiency can impair fertility and increase the risk of miscarriage.

Mood Swings and Anxiety: Progesterone has calming effects on the central nervous system, and deficiency can lead to mood swings, anxiety, and depression.

Insomnia and Disrupted Sleep Patterns: Progesterone promotes relaxation and sleep, and deficiency can result in insomnia, difficulty falling asleep, or disrupted sleep patterns.

These effects underscore the critical importance of maintaining a delicate balance between estrogen and progesterone for optimal reproductive health and overall well-being.

Endocrine Disrupting Chemicals (EDCs)

Endocrine Disrupting Chemicals (EDCs) are environmental toxins that have gained significant attention due to their potential to disrupt hormonal balance in humans and even wildlife. These chemicals interfere with the endocrine system, which is responsible for regulating various physiological processes by producing and secreting hormones. EDCs can mimic, block, or interfere with the body's natural hormones, leading to hormone imbalances and adverse health effects.

Research has shown that exposure to EDCs is associated with a wide range of health issues, including reproductive disorders, developmental abnormalities, metabolic disorders, and certain types of cancer. In women, EDCs have been linked to menstrual irregularities, infertility, PCOS, endometriosis, and breast cancer.

The discovery of EDCs dates back several decades. In the 1940s and 1950s, scientists first observed adverse reproductive effects in wildlife exposed to industrial chemicals such as dichlorodiphenyltrichloroethane (DDT) and polychlorinated biphenyls (PCBs) which is further explored below. Subsequent research identified similar effects in humans, leading to increased scrutiny of chemicals in the environment and their potential impact on hormone systems.

Since then, numerous studies have investigated the mechanisms by which EDCs disrupt hormonal balance. These chemicals can exert their effects through various pathways, including binding to hormone receptors, altering hormone synthesis or metabolism, and interfering with signalling pathways involved in hormone regulation. Additionally, exposure to EDCs during critical periods of development, such as fetal development and puberty, can have long-lasting effects on reproductive and metabolic health.

EDCs are pervasive in the environment and can be found in everyday products such as plastics, pesticides, personal care products, and flame retardants. They enter the body through ingestion, inhalation, and skin contact, and can accumulate in adipose tissue and other organs over time. Despite efforts to regulate and reduce exposure to EDCs, their widespread presence poses a significant public health challenge.

One group of EDCs that is particularly concerning for women's health are those that mimic estrogen, known as 'Estrogenic EDCs'. These chemicals can bind to estrogen receptors in the body, thereby exerting estrogenic effects and disrupting normal hormonal function.

Some examples of estrogenic EDCs include:

1. **Bisphenol A (BPA):** Found in plastics, food and beverage containers, thermal paper receipts, and dental sealants, BPA is a well-known estrogenic chemical that has been linked to reproductive and developmental abnormalities.

2. **Phthalates:** These chemicals are commonly used as plasticisers in various consumer products, including cosmetics, personal care products, vinyl flooring, and food packaging. Phthalates have been associated with adverse effects on reproductive health, including altered menstrual cycles, reduced fertility, and pregnancy complications.

3. **Parabens:** Widely used as preservatives in cosmetics, skincare products, and pharmaceuticals, parabens have estrogenic properties and can disrupt hormone signalling in the body.

4. **Fragrances:** Often used in perfumes, cosmetics, cleaning products, and air fresheners, many synthetic fragrances contain

chemicals that can act as endocrine disruptors. These chemicals can mimic estrogen and interfere with hormone function, potentially leading to reproductive and developmental issues.

5. **Triclosan:** Commonly found in antibacterial soaps, toothpaste, and some cosmetics, triclosan is an antimicrobial agent with estrogenic effects. It has been linked to hormone disruption and could contribute to antibiotic resistance and environmental pollution.

6. **Glyphosate**: Commonly found in herbicides like Roundup, which is widely used in agriculture and gardening, including here in Australia, glyphosate has been suggested to act as an endocrine-disrupting chemical (EDC) with potential estrogenic effects. Some studies have indicated that glyphosate can bind to estrogen receptors, potentially disrupting the body's hormone regulation. Its ability to mimic or interfere with estrogen signalling has raised concerns about its impact on reproductive health and hormone balance.

Minimising exposure to Endocrine Disrupting Chemicals (EDCs)

Minimising exposure to EDCs is essential for protecting our hormonal health. I know this information can be overwhelming if you're learning about it for the first time, but there are simple steps you can take that, over time, can make a huge difference in reducing your toxic load. Fortunately, there are several practical strategies that you can adopt to lower their exposure to these harmful chemicals.

Choose Natural Products: opt for natural personal care products that are free of phthalates, parabens, and other known EDCs. Look for labels that indicate products are "phthalate-free," "paraben-free," or "fragrance-free." Consider making your own natural skincare and cleaning products using simple ingredients like baking soda, vinegar, and essential oils.

Avoid Plastics: Minimise the use of plastic containers, especially those containing bisphenol A (BPA) and other estrogenic chemicals. Instead, choose glass or stainless-steel containers for food storage and avoid heating food in plastic containers, as this can leach chemicals into the food. When purchasing canned foods, look for brands that use BPA-free lining.

Silicone is a safer alternative to plastics, particularly for food storage and preparation, as it does not contain harmful chemicals like BPA or phthalates. Its high heat resistance (from -40°F to 450°F) makes it safe for use in microwaves and ovens, reducing the risk of chemical leaching. Silicone works well with glass and stainless-steel containers, creating airtight seals and minimizing the need for single-use plastics. While not biodegradable, its durability makes it a more sustainable choice compared to traditional plastics.

Eat Organic: Choose organic produce whenever possible to reduce exposure to pesticides, which can contain EDCs. Washing fruits and vegetables thoroughly can also help remove pesticide residues. Additionally, opt for hormone-free and organic dairy products and meat to avoid potential exposure to hormones used in conventional livestock production.

Cook Safely: Use safe cookware options such as stainless steel, cast iron, or ceramic instead of non-stick cookware, which may contain perfluoroalkyl substances (PFAS) that can leach into food. Avoid using plastic utensils and silicone cookware, especially at high temperatures.

Filter Your Water: Invest in a high-quality water filter to remove contaminants such as chlorine, fluoride, and heavy metals from your tap water. Some water filters can also remove EDCs like phthalates and bisphenols.

Detoxify Naturally: Support your body's natural detoxification processes by incorporating antioxidant-rich foods into your diet, such as fruits, vegetables, nuts, seeds, and green tea. Consider engaging in detoxifying practices like sauna sessions, dry brushing, and regular exercise to help eliminate toxins from the body.

Educate Yourself: Stay informed about potential sources of EDC exposure and take proactive steps to minimise risk. Read labels carefully when purchasing household products, cosmetics, and food packaging, and choose brands that prioritise safety and transparency.

Hot tip: If a product contains ingredients such as parabens, phthalates, or triclosan, it's best to avoid it, as these chemicals are commonly associated with endocrine disruption and potential health risks discussed above. Instead, opt for products labelled as "paraben-free," "phthalate-free," or "natural" to reduce exposure.

By implementing these strategies gradually and making informed choices about the products you use and the foods you consume, you can significantly reduce your exposure to EDCs and protect your hormonal health for the long term.

Chapter 4
Sisterhood, The Red Tent and the Moon

"Secret women's business" historically encompassed cultural taboos and segregation—but it also represented a time when women would share wisdom, support, and teach each other about menstruation and reproductive health. In many traditional societies, elder women would guide younger girls through the changes of puberty, passing down knowledge about their bodies in a communal and supportive environment. This positive aspect of secret women's business fostered a sense of sisterhood and empowerment, as women helped each other navigate the complexities of their health.

As societies modernised and became more industrialised, the practice of openly discussing menstruation diminished significantly. The rise of Victorian modesty and the increasing medicalisation of women's bodies led to a shift where menstruation became a topic of silence and even shame. Many women who grew up during this time recall not being informed about their periods, leading to confusion and fear when they first began menstruating. It's heartbreaking to hear stories of young girls who, unprepared and uninformed, thought they were dying when they first started bleeding. This lack of communication and education around such a fundamental aspect of women's health left many feeling isolated and embarrassed.

Thankfully, we are now witnessing a significant shift in how society approaches menstrual education and women's health. The silence is being broken, and there is a growing movement towards open, honest, and positive conversations about menstruation. This change is driven by the efforts of educators, activists, and health professionals who recognise the importance of demystifying menstruation and providing accurate information to everyone, regardless of gender.

Educational programs in schools are starting to include comprehensive information about menstruation and reproductive health, ensuring that adolescents understand these natural processes. Social media campaigns and advocacy groups are working tirelessly to end period poverty and stigma, emphasising that access to menstrual products and information is a fundamental right. The resurgence of community-focused initiatives mirrors the supportive environment of the past, where knowledge about menstruation was shared and celebrated rather than hidden.

This shift is incredibly gratifying, as it represents a return to the positive aspects of secret women's business—where women support, educate, and empower each other. Today, men are also being included in these conversations, fostering a more inclusive and informed society that respects and supports women's health and well-being. The transformation from secrecy and shame to openness and empowerment is a testament to the progress we are making towards a more equitable and understanding world.

Sacred Spaces During Menstruation

Indigenous cultures worldwide have traditions of women gathering in sacred spaces during menstruation or other significant life events. These gatherings often involve rituals, storytelling, and support networks among women.

The Red Tent represents a sanctuary in where women would gather during menstruation, childbirth, and other significant life events. It provided a sacred space for women to bond, share experiences, and receive support from one another. The ritual of women bleeding together on a new moon and ovulating on a full moon is deeply significant. This practice not only reflects the interconnectedness between women's menstrual cycles and the lunar cycle but also underscores the ancient recognition of this connection in various cultures worldwide.

The story of The Red Tent draws inspiration from various cultures and historical contexts where women have sought refuge and companionship in sacred spaces. While the specific narrative is a fictional creation, it is influenced by historical practices and traditions that have resonated throughout time.

Biblical references also contribute to the narrative of the Red Tent, particularly the story of Dinah, daughter of Jacob and Leah, mentioned briefly in the Book of Genesis. Anita Diamant's novel "The Red Tent" fictionalises Dinah's life and imagines the experiences of women in biblical times. Through her storytelling, Diamant brings to life the sisterhood and resilience of women as they navigate the challenges of ancient society.

In exploring the significance of the Red Tent, we acknowledge the contributions of Anita Diamant and other writers who have brought this concept to life through their storytelling.

Hawaiian Menstruation Culture

In traditional Hawaiian culture, menstruation was viewed as a natural and powerful expression of womanhood, closely tied to spiritual energy and the cycles of nature. While detailed records of specific menstrual practices are limited, the broader cultural beliefs reflect a respect for the menstrual cycle, recognising it as a source of wisdom and a deep connection to the natural rhythms of the earth and moon.

One important concept in Hawaiian culture is Kapu, or sacred prohibitions, which governed many aspects of daily life, including menstruation[2]. During their menstrual cycles, women were believed to possess a heightened spiritual energy, known as mana, a form of spiritual power. To protect both themselves and the community from the intense power of mana, women observed specific Kapu related to cleanliness, seclusion, and spiritual practice.

---

[2] *The information about menstrual cycle traditions in Hawaiian culture is based on historical accounts, cultural studies, and ethnographic research conducted by scholars and anthropologists who have studied Hawaiian society and traditions.*

Women would often retreat to designated hale pe'a (menstrual huts) during their periods. These huts were typically located away from the main living areas, providing women with privacy and a place to rest and reflect. While in the hale pe'a, women practiced self-care, reconnected with their bodies, and participated in rituals to honour their menstrual cycles. Although specific details of these rituals are not well-documented, the practice of seclusion and reflection underscores the importance of this time in the cycle.

Hawaiian culture was deeply connected to the natural world, particularly the cycles of the moon (mahina) and the sea (moana), both of which were seen as related to fertility and the female reproductive system. The moon was believed to influence the rhythms of life, including the menstrual cycle, aligning with Hawaiian respect for cyclical living.

Women used oli (chants) and pule (prayers) during menstruation to seek protection, balance, and connection to the natural world. These spiritual practices likely helped women navigate this time with reverence for their bodies and the cycles of nature.

Overall, these cultural practices reflect the deep spiritual connection Hawaiians had with nature and the body's cycles, recognising the importance of honouring the cyclical nature of life and maintaining balance between the individual and the natural world

Period Stigma

While the Red Tent and menstrual huts symbolise spaces of empowerment and solidarity for women, it's essential to acknowledge the dark side of these historical practices. Throughout history, women have faced dire consequences due to inadequate hygiene or societal taboos surrounding menstruation. In some cultures, women were confined to menstrual huts or caves during their periods, where they were isolated and lacked access to proper sanitation.

Tragically, there have been instances where women have died due to complications arising from these conditions, highlighting the urgent need to challenge harmful beliefs and practices surrounding menstruation.

However, amidst these challenges, we praise all women who have worked tirelessly to help change these harmful beliefs and practices. Their advocacy, education, and activism have been instrumental in raising awareness about menstruation and advocating for the rights and dignity of menstruating individuals.

By challenging stigma, promoting access to menstrual hygiene products, and fostering open conversations about menstruation, these women have contributed to creating a more inclusive and supportive environment for all. Their efforts have paved the way for greater acceptance, understanding, and respect for menstruating individuals, empowering women to embrace their bodies and menstrual cycles with pride and confidence.

The word "period" itself derives from the Greek word "periodos," meaning "cycle" or "recurring time." Historically, menstruation has been shrouded in misconceptions and stigma, leading to the perception of menstrual bleeding as a pathological condition. In ancient times, menstruation was often associated with impurity or illness, and menstrual bleeding was thought to be a symptom of a periodic disease afflicting women.

These erroneous beliefs perpetuated harmful attitudes towards menstruating individuals, reinforcing societal norms that marginalised and stigmatised women based on their reproductive biology. It's crucial to recognise the historical context surrounding menstruation and challenge the stigma and misinformation that continues to affect women's health today.

The Symbolism of the Moon and Menstrual Cycles

In traditional societies, the moon has been seen as a symbol of femininity, fertility, and renewal. Women would come together during the new moon, a time for darkness and reflection, to honour their periods and take part in cleansing and renewal rituals. This special time helped them connect with themselves and each other.

Ovulation during the full moon represented a time of brightness and energy, marking the peak of fertility and the potential for new life.

This connection not only provided a natural rhythm for gatherings and shared experiences but also created a sense of empowerment and support among women.

In today's world, with artificial lighting and changes in our lifestyles, this link between the menstrual cycle and the moon has become weaker and is often ignore

White Moon and Red Moon

Understanding the concepts of the White Moon and Red Moon cycles offers fascinating insight into the ancient belief systems surrounding the menstrual cycle and its connection to the phases of the moon.

These concepts were notably discussed by author Miranda Gray in her book *"Red Moon"*, which explores the spiritual significance of menstruation and its connection to lunar phases.

We can draw inspiration from ancient cultures that observed the moon's influence on life, such as in agriculture and fertility, they also serve as metaphors for how menstrual cycles align with different energies associated with the moon.

While not scientifically necessary for managing your hormone health, these archetypes provide an interesting lens through which to explore the cyclical nature of women's bodies and their potential alignment with lunar rhythms.

White Moon – Menstruation Aligns with the New Moon

The White Moon phase occurs when menstruation aligns with the new moon (when the least amount of moonlight is reaching the earth). During this time, women often experience a sense of inner cleansing and renewal. It invites deep reflection and contemplation, allowing for the release of old patterns and the setting of new intentions. Women may find serenity and peace as they embrace this opportunity for personal growth and transformation.

Spiritually, the White Moon phase represents alignment with higher consciousness and spiritual truth. Women often feel more connected to their spiritual practices—such as meditation, prayer, or ritual—as they seek guidance and insight from the divine. This phase creates a sacred space for inner exploration and a deeper connection to one's innate wisdom and essence.

Red Moon – Menstruation during a Full Moon

In contrast, the Red Moon phase is associated with menstruation during the full moon. This phase is characterised by heightened energy, passion, and emotional expression. As the moon reaches its full brightness, women may feel a surge of vitality and empowerment, fully embracing their feminine strength.

Emotionally, the Red Moon phase encourages courage and boldness, prompting women to express themselves authentically. It is a time to embrace desires and pursue creative endeavours with enthusiasm. Many women feel more outgoing and assertive during this phase, tapping into their inherent strength and resilience.

Syncing your Menstrual Cycle with the Moon

Syncing your menstrual cycle with the moon phases is a practice that involves attuning to the natural rhythms of the lunar cycle and your own body's cycle. While syncing your cycle with the moon is not necessary for hormone health, some women find it to be a meaningful way to connect with nature and their own bodies. You may discover that you're already naturally synced with the moon, or you might want to try aligning your cycle with the lunar phases.

If so, here are some tips to help you sync your cycle with the moon phases:

- Tracking your menstrual cycle and the phases of the moon to identify any patterns or correlations.

- Setting intentions or performing rituals during the new moon or full moon to align with the energy of the lunar phase.

- Engaging in practices such as meditation, journaling, or yoga to connect with your inner self and cultivate awareness of your menstrual cycle and the moon phases.

- Spending time in nature and observing the moon's cycles to deepen your connection to the natural world and the cosmic rhythms that influence us all.

An example of a new moon ritual could be setting intentions to harness the energy of new beginnings and fresh starts.

New Moon Ritual Example:

1. **Create a Sacred Space:** Light a candle and set the mood.
2. **Write Your Intentions:** Reflect on what you want to manifest and write it down.
3. **Meditate:** Visualise your intentions as you meditate.
4. **Release:** Fold the paper and place it in water or bury it to symbolise planting your intentions.

Mantra:
"I release the past and embrace new beginnings. I am open to all that the universe has to offer."

Full Moon Ritual Example:

1. **Gather Supplies:** Prepare water and salt for purification.
2. **Reflect:** Acknowledge achievements since the new moon.
3. **Release Ceremony:** Write down what you want to let go of and burn or place it in saltwater.
4. **Gratitude:** Express gratitude for your journey.

Mantra:
"I release what no longer serves me and welcome clarity. I am grateful for the journey ahead."

Incorporating seed cycling into your diet having Phase 1 seeds during a new moon and Phase 2 seeds during a full moon can also help align your cycle with the moon phases.

Whether or not you believe in the spiritual significance of lunar menstruation, honouring your body's natural rhythms and embracing your menstrual cycle as a sacred and integral part of your being can promote greater self-awareness, empowerment, and well-being.

The connection between menstrual cycles, sisterhood, and lunar rhythms extend beyond cultural practices and spiritual beliefs—it also holds significance in the realm of personal growth and self-discovery. Through practices such as journaling, meditation, and ritual, we can harness the power of our menstrual cycles to enhance creativity, intuition, and spiritual connection

.

Chapter 5
Cyclical Rhythms and The Menstrual Cycle

Let us now delve into the profound interconnectedness between the cyclical rhythms observed in nature and those inherent in the menstrual cycle. Just as the natural world exhibits a rhythmic pattern of growth, decline, and renewal, so too does the rhythms within the female body. This information may be entirely new to you, and like me, you may have spent most of your life viewing your menstrual cycle solely as your period, never encountering the terms "follicular phase or luteal phase" or understanding these intricate rhythms and the significance of them.

Life unfolds in cycles, deeply intertwined with the rhythms of the natural world. From the waxing and waning of the moon to the shifting dance of the seasons and the perpetual cycle of life and death, these patterns weave through the very fabric of existence, guiding the ebb and flow of all living things.

Scientific understanding confirms the presence of cyclical patterns in nature, from the changing seasons to the rhythmic orbits, the regular, predictable paths that objects like planets, moons, and stars follow as they move through space.

As I embrace cyclical living, it serves as a beautiful, constant reminder of my unity with nature. By attuning to these rhythms with my menstrual cycle, I deepen my understanding of my body and connect with a wisdom that speaks to the inherent harmony between my body and nature.

Phases of the Menstrual Cycle

Every woman has her own unique experience of her menstrual cycle, yet there is a shared pattern among the phases, with each phase having its own distinct characteristics and functions.

These phases include menstruation, follicular phase, ovulation, and the luteal phase. Together, they form a dynamic and interconnected cycle that reflects the inherent wisdom of the female body and its capacity for birthing, regeneration and renewal.

At the heart of this cyclical journey lies the hormonal messengers within our bodies, orchestrating the phases of our menstrual cycle with precision and purpose. From the emergence of a follicle in the ovary to the shedding of the uterine lining, each phase of the menstrual cycle is governed by a delicate interplay of hormonal signals and physiological changes.

The Seasons and The Menstrual Cycle

Let's further explore the parallels between the cyclical rhythms observed in nature and the phases of the menstrual cycle. One striking comparison is the association between the seasons and the menstrual cycle.

The cyclical changes in nature, such as the changing seasons, can be seen as reflections of the cyclical changes within the human body, including the menstrual cycle. The four seasons—spring, summer, autumn, and winter—are metaphorically linked to the different phases of the menstrual cycle: menstruation, follicular phase, ovulation, and luteal phase, respectively.

Menstrual Phase – Release

The follicular phase is the first half of your cycle, beginning with the start of your period and lasting until ovulation. The menstrual phase, often referred to as our inner Winter, marks the beginning of our bleed which can last between 3-7 days. During this phase, your hormones are at their lowest as the lining of your uterus, the endometrium sheds.

Cyclical Rhythms and The Menstrual Cycle

Your menstrual phase is a time of release, introspection, and rest, much like the quiet and contemplative nature of winter. As your uterine lining sheds in preparation for a new cycle of growth and regeneration, it can represent a natural process of release and purification.

For some women, the energy of the menstrual phase can be a huge relief as the tumultuous premenstrual energies cease, bringing some inner peace. Giving ourselves permission to rest and relax during the menstrual phase allows us to dream our dreams into existence, check in with our souls, and heal and restore our physical bodies.

Sadly, when we don't stop, and when our modern world doesn't allow this, we lose out on the restoring and healing energy of this phase. By being still, resting, and daydreaming, we fill ourselves with love and gain clarity on our true goals and dreams.

Embracing my menstrual phase has been a transformative journey for me. In the past, my menstrual phase was overshadowed by inconvenience and annoyance. I used to resort to using the pill to skip periods to avoid dealing with my bleed. However, as I've grown and learned more about the phases of my menstrual cycle and the hormonal changes that accompany them, I've come to cherish and welcome this phase each month.

Now, I see it as a time of shedding and releasing both physically and mentally letting go of built-up stress, negative self-talk, and feelings of doubt or frustration that may have surfaced in the previous cycle. It's a time for me to set goals, to dream about what I want for my life and the month ahead. I use this time to ask for what I want and let go of what is no longer serving me, to put my intentions out into the universe. Rather than viewing it as a burden, I see it as an opportunity for growth and self-care.

I've embraced period undies and find comfort in staying at home during mt bleed, allowing myself the space and time to fully experience the shedding and renewal that comes with it. I also feel incredibly creative during this phase. I enjoy channelling this creativity into writing and developing ideas. I love arts and crafts activities with my kids, I can easily find joy and inspiration in the process of creation while in my menstrual phase.

Nutrition for the Menstrual Phase

During the menstrual phase, prioritising nutrient-rich foods can help you optimise this phase and alleviate common symptoms such as cramps, fatigue, bloating, and mood swings. Some recommended nutrients and foods during this time include:

Iron-rich foods: Since menstruation can lead to a loss of iron through blood loss, consuming iron-rich foods such as meats, liver, poultry, fish, beans, lentils and spinach can help replenish iron stores and prevent fatigue and weakness.

Magnesium: Magnesium is known for its role in muscle relaxation and mood regulation. Foods high in magnesium include dark leafy greens (like spinach and kale), nuts and seeds (such as almonds and pumpkin seeds), whole grains, and legumes.

Seed Cycling Phase 1: Helps regulate estrogen levels, which are crucial during menstruation. By promoting healthy estrogen levels, seed cycling can contribute to overall hormonal balance and pave the way for optimal menstrual health.

Vitamin B6: Vitamin B6 has been shown to help alleviate symptoms of PMS, including mood swings and bloating. Foods rich in vitamin B6 include chickpeas, salmon, chicken, bananas and potatoes.

Omega-3 Fatty Acids: Omega-3 fatty acids have anti-inflammatory properties and can help reduce menstrual cramps and inflammation. Sources of Omega-3s include fatty fish (such as salmon, mackerel, and sardines), flaxseeds, chia seeds, walnuts, and hemp seeds.

Calcium: Calcium is important for muscle and nerve function and can help reduce menstrual cramps. Yoghurt, kefir and cheese are rich sources of calcium, as are leafy greens like kale and collard greens.

During my menstrual phase, I've discovered the power of nourishing foods to support my body's needs. One of my favourite rituals during this time is making liver pate and enjoying it on sourdough bread. The rich flavours and nutrient density of liver provide me with a sense of grounding and vitality that I find incredibly comforting.

Additionally, I've incorporated warm, nourishing foods into my diet, which helps alleviate any discomfort or fatigue I experience. One of my go-to treats during this phase is my Seed Cycle Brownie Mix, made with raw cacao and packed with the nutrients from flax and pumpkin seeds. Not only does it satisfy my cravings, but it also provides me with essential nutrients to support hormonal balance.

> **Summary:** This phase is about introspection and creativity, where the groundwork for the future and dreams are laid. During the menstrual phase, gentle exercises such as walking, restorative yoga, Pilates, swimming, Tai Chi and stretching help promote relaxation.
>
> **Rital:** Inspired by Red Moon by Amanda Grey, you can acknowledge and honour your menstrual phase by placing a small bowl or empty vase on a visible shelf or counter, serving as a reminder to cherish this time of release.

Follicular Phase – Awaken

Your "inner Spring," follicular phase or pre-ovulation, starts right after your bleed ends. As your body moves into this refreshing phase, follicle-stimulating hormone (FSH) increases, promoting the growth and development of follicles in your ovaries. This is a time of renewal and rising energy, as your body prepares for ovulation.

This phase embodies a sense of renewal and potential, mirroring the rejuvenating essence of Spring in nature. Just as the earth awakens from dormancy, bursting forth with vitality and the promise of new beginnings, the phase heralds the body's readiness for the possibility of conception and the creation of new life.

The energy during the pre-ovulation phase brings a sense of self and excitement about being alive. This phase is characterised by a surge of energy, enthusiasm, and a zest for life. The phase begins as we awaken from the menstrual hibernation phase, and for many women, this is a time of vitality and opportunity. We can feel reborn, our sexual desire may grow, and we are filled with self-belief, ready to take on plans and actions.

You may find that with each phase comes a different thinking pattern, our thinking becomes more logical and focused. We find it easier to concentrate and are more likely to step out of our comfort zones. Certain tasks may feel easier and faster, making this the ideal time of the month to start new projects, stay up late working, and make things happen. We know what we want and how to achieve it.

Many women (myself included) wish to stay in this phase throughout their entire cycle, especially in our modern world, as we can work longer, harder, and faster, feeling less emotional and stronger. Yet, when we suppress the other phases, we lose the unique gifts they have to offer.

After my period ends, I experience a surge of energy and motivation, feeling awakened and eager to tackle everything on my to-do list. However, I notice that my perfectionism intensifies during this phase, leading to frustration as I strive for unattainable levels of perfection in various aspects of my life. Recognising this pattern allows me to acknowledge that it's my pre-ovulation phase. Instead of becoming overwhelmed, I use this time to prioritise tasks that I've been putting off and focus on getting the hard work done. Grounding myself and staying mindful helps me channel my heightened energy into productive activities, making the most of this phase's vitality and drive.

Nutrition for the Follicular Phase

During the follicular phase, nutrition plays a crucial role in supporting the body's increased energy levels and metabolic activity. You may find that your appetite naturally decreases during this phase, and intermittent fasting with longer windows of 14 to 16 hours can be beneficial for some women. This approach allows your body to tap into fat stores for energy and promotes cellular repair and renewal.

Additionally, focusing on nutrient-dense foods such as leafy greens, whole grains, lean proteins, and healthy fats provides essential vitamins and minerals to support hormone balance and overall well-being during this phase. Incorporating plenty of hydrating foods like fruits and vegetables can also help maintain optimal hydration levels, supporting your body's increased energy expenditure and metabolic needs.

Incorporating The Seed Cycle™ Phase 1 can help support hormone balance and prepare the body for ovulation. Healthy estrogen levels during this phase are essential as they lead to healthy progesterone levels later in the cycle.

> **Summary**: Energy levels rise, making it an ideal time for action and productivity. You may like to make a list of all the things you want to get done in this phase. Focus on nourishing foods and mindful eating. Incorporate intense workouts like strength training, cardio, and outdoor activities to leverage your increased energy and motivation. Choose exercises that make you feel strong and energised.
>
> **Rital:** After menstruation, display a small vase of white flowers on a shelf or counter where you can see it to acknowledge and honour your follicular, pre-ovulation phase.

Ovulation - Peak

Ovulation, known as our inner Summer, signifies the midpoint of the menstrual cycle, typically occurring around halfway through. It represents the pinnacle of fertility, marked by the release of a mature egg from the ovary, poised to journey down the fallopian tube in anticipation of fertilisation. Ovulation is sparked by a surge in luteinising hormone (LH), prompting the follicle to rupture and liberate the egg. This phase is often accompanied by a surge in energy and vitality, mirroring the vibrant and dynamic essence of summer in nature.

Additionally, heightened libido and sexual desire are commonly experienced during ovulation, aligning with the season's theme of passion and abundance. Just as summer brings forth an abundance of life and growth, ovulation symbolises the peak of fertility and the potential for new beginnings.

During this time, we can feel gentler and let go of many of the projects from the follicular phase. It's a period of strength, love, and groundedness, where we can listen, help others, and feel compassionate. We can create the best conditions for others to grow. In this caring and peaceful phase, our feeling mind becomes dominant. We are naturally open and accepting, and it feels good to be loving and nurturing.

At ovulation, I feel at my peak in both libido and vitality. I feel sparkly and bright, like a magnet drawing energy and opportunities toward me. It's a time when I find it easy to speak, and I love engaging in workshops, podcasts, interviews, and social activities. For me, ovulation is when I feel most at ease with myself, using this time to make brave decisions. Whether it's reaching out to someone I admire for collaboration or saying the difficult word "no" to something that doesn't align with my values, ovulation empowers me to take charge. Reflecting on this, I can't help but feel a bit cheated by the time I spent on the pill because I missed out on experiencing the peak of ovulation.

During ovulation, exercises that promote energy, strength, and flexibility can be particularly beneficial. Activities like strength training, yoga, and Pilates are great choices. These exercises help to maintain energy levels, boost mood, and support overall physical well-being during this phase. Additionally, incorporating activities that you enjoy and find invigorating can enhance the positive effects of exercise during ovulation.

Nutrition for the Ovulation Phase

Focus on foods that support liver function and hormone balance as estrogen levels peak and are about to decline. Incorporate nutrient-rich options like leafy greens, whole grains, lean proteins, avocados, nuts, and seeds. These foods provide essential nutrients to aid hormone production and regulate detox pathways. Switch to The Seed Cycle™ Phase 2 to support ovulation and move smoothly through your luteal phase.

During ovulation, I find great joy in spending time in the kitchen, preparing meals for myself and my loved ones. This phase brings a heightened sense of energy and creativity, allowing me to explore more complex recipes and try new culinary adventures. Cooking becomes a form of self-expression and nourishment, as I pour my creativity and care into the dishes I create. It is a time of abundance and vitality, and I embrace the opportunity to savour the flavours and delights of cooking during this phase of my cycle.

> **Summary:** Enjoy romance and nurturing relationships as well your emotional depth and empathy which can feel heightened during this phase.

Rital: Welcome ovulation by placing a small vase of pink flowers on a shelf or counter where you can see it. This gentle reminder helps us embrace the loving, nurturing energy of this phase.

Premenstrual Luteal Phase – Reflection

During the luteal or premenstrual phase, our bodies transition after ovulation, moving towards the next menstrual cycle. It's like our inner Autumn, a time for reflection and change. After ovulation, estrogen levels dip before rising again briefly, only to decline towards the end of the cycle. Meanwhile, the follicle that released the egg transforms into the corpus luteum, a temporary structure that produces progesterone. This hormone plays a crucial role in preparing the uterus for a potential pregnancy by thickening the uterine lining. If fertilisation doesn't occur, progesterone levels decrease, triggering the start of menstruation.

The luteal phase brings change into our lives, sometimes gently and sometimes with force. It can bring both high and low energies. Deep needs that have not been given attention can come to the forefront, and our subconscious mind becomes dominant, making it harder to think logically. This time can be used to clear away old patterns as we travel further into ourselves. We often fight our premenstrual phase and our cyclical nature to fit in and perform in the modern world, but embracing the luteal phase can lead to profound personal growth and transformation.

This phase often feels turbulent, and I notice I am overly critical of myself and others. However, I have come to understand that these feelings are not only normal but also serve as opportunities for growth and self-awareness. By journaling and reflecting on my thoughts and emotions during the luteal phase, I can gain insight into what needs changing and release any pent-up tension or negativity, paving the way for a more balanced and harmonious menstrual phase.

During this phase, I find EFT Tapping incredibly helpful in acknowledging and accepting the emotions that arise. Here are also some journaling prompts that may help you navigate the luteal phase:

What emotions am I experiencing during this phase?

Are there any recurring patterns or themes in my thoughts and emotions during the luteal phase?

What activities or practices bring me comfort and relaxation during this phase?

How can I nurture and support myself physically, emotionally, and mentally during the luteal phase?

What insights or realisations have I gained about myself during previous luteal phases?

How can I cultivate gratitude and appreciation for my body's natural rhythms and cycles?

Are there any adjustments or changes I can make to my routine to better support myself during this phase?

Nature and sunlight are essential for me throughout all phases of my menstrual cycle, but particularly during my luteal phase. I find that spending time outdoors, soaking up the natural sunlight, helps me navigate the emotional and physical changes that come with this phase. Focus on exercises like strength training, yoga, Pilates, walking, swimming, and cycling to support your body's natural rhythms and energy levels.

I make it a practice to wake up with the sunrise and spend at least 10 minutes outside, soaking in the serene surroundings and feeling grounded for the day ahead. On average, experts recommend spending at least 10 to 15 minutes in the morning sunlight to reap its benefits. This is because morning sunlight contains a higher concentration of vitamin D, crucial for bone health, immune system function, and mood regulation. Additionally, exposure to morning sunlight can help regulate our circadian rhythm, leading to better sleep patterns.

In the evening, I love watching the sunset, enjoying the beautiful colours and feeling peaceful. These moments outdoors help me find balance and serenity during this reflective time of the month.

Nutrition for the Luteal Phase

During the luteal phase, the body's energy requirements often increase due to hormonal fluctuations, particularly the dominance of progesterone. As a result, consuming an adequate amount of complex carbohydrates becomes crucial to fuel metabolism and support overall well-being during this phase. Carbohydrates serve as the primary source of energy for the body, providing glucose that cells use for various physiological functions, including hormone production and metabolism.

Additionally, carbohydrates help regulate serotonin levels in the brain, which can contribute to mood stability. Therefore, including complex carbohydrates from whole grains, fruits, and vegetables in the diet can help maintain energy levels, support hormonal balance, and promote emotional well-being throughout the luteal phase.

In addition to carbohydrates, incorporating The Seed Cycle™ Phase 2 into your diet during the luteal phase can further support hormonal balance. These seeds can help modulate estrogen levels and promote detoxification pathways in the body, aiding in the elimination of excess hormones and toxins.

Coffee sensitivity can vary depending on individual hormone levels and responses. Generally, during the luteal phase, which occurs after ovulation and before menstruation, some individuals may experience increased sensitivity to caffeine due to hormonal fluctuations. This heightened sensitivity may be attributed to changes in progesterone levels, which can affect how the body metabolises caffeine. However, individual responses may vary, and some people may not notice significant differences in coffee sensitivity throughout their menstrual cycle.

> **Summary:** Finally, a period of refection and taking what you need, recognising the importance of replenishing your own reserves. The warmth of the sun and the beauty of nature have a calming effect on my mind and body, easing any tension or discomfort I may be experiencing.
>
> **Rital:** Greet the luteal phase by placing a small vase of dark flowers on a shelf or bench where you can see them,

symbolising your acknowledgment and acceptance of this transformative and introspective time.

I want to acknowledge that despite my best intentions and knowledge, there are times when I struggle to maintain my health and wellness practices and rituals. Life can throw us curveballs, and external events can impact our energy, hearts, and souls. During these challenging times, let's make a commitment to be gentle with ourselves and avoid self-judgment. Let's practice self-compassion and use these moments as opportunities for reflection. I often remind myself that I'm fortunate to have another cycle ahead, offering a chance to try again. When I have a month where I don't prioritise self-care, nutrition and movement, I feel its effects. For me it serves as a powerful reminder of the importance of honouring my health and my cycle and reminds me how much these practices truly benefit me.

Cycles with Irregular Periods, on the Pill, during Pregnancy or Menopause

For individuals who are on hormonal contraceptives such as the Pill, have irregular cycles, are pregnant, during menopause, or have undergone a hysterectomy, syncing with the natural menstrual phases may not align.

In such cases, aligning with the moon phases can serve as a dominant rhythm. By observing the waxing and waning of the moon, you can attune to the natural cycles of the lunar calendar, fostering a deeper connection with nature's rhythms and harnessing its energy for their own well-being.

Additionally, understanding the phases of the menstrual cycle and their associated energy and nutrient requirements can be beneficial for individuals planning to transition off hormonal contraceptives in the future. Further exploration of these concepts will be discussed in the following chapters, offering insights into how to navigate and embrace the interplay between the menstrual and lunar cycles for holistic health and wellness.

By honouring and attuning to cyclical rhythms, we can tap into a deeper connection with ourselves and the natural world, fostering a sense of harmony, balance, and health. Through mindfulness and awareness, we can harness the wisdom of cyclical living to support our health, vitality, and growth.

Introducing Kids to Understanding Menstrual Cycles

I believe that a key step toward breaking the stigma and misconceptions surrounding menstruation is to educate my kids in a positive and empowering way. Introducing the topic through a fictional story can make it more relatable and set the stage for clear, informative discussions. This approach helps create a foundation of understanding, reducing negativity and promoting open conversations.

While researching, I noticed that much of the information available emphasises symptoms like bloating, PMS, and the discomfort often associated with periods. Instead, I choose to approach menstrual education for kids from a more positive perspective, focusing on the natural and empowering aspects of the cycle. These symptoms, while common, shouldn't be considered the standard, and I prefer to share a balanced view without focusing on discomfort. This helps frame menstruation as a healthy, natural process rather than something to dread or feel embarrassed about.

A Story to Begin With

You could introduce menstruation by saying: "As you grow into a woman, your body is becoming ready to have a baby. Every month or so, your ovaries start releasing hormones that cause the lining of your uterus (the special place where a baby can grow) to build up because it is ready for a fertilised egg."

The Story: The Uterus Decorators

This story is inspired by the wonderful Kim Morrison, who shared with me a heartfelt tale her friend Faye told her daughter.

> "A uterus a is the special place in a female body where a baby can grow. Imagine your uterus is like a baby's bedroom. When you have a baby, it lives and grows in this room for nine months. Every month, a special team of decorators receives a mission to prepare a beautiful room for a baby. They paint the

walls in lovely colours, hang up pretty pictures, set up a cozy cot, and lay out the tiniest, cutest baby clothes.

These decorators work very hard, making everything perfect in preparation for a baby. But some months, the baby doesn't arrive, so when that happens, the decorators take everything down and clean up the room. They carefully take down the pictures, pack away the cot, and fold up the baby clothes. This cleanup process is what we know as a period.

So, having a period is just like the decorators tiding up and getting ready for the next cycle. It's a natural and important part of life, keeping everything in perfect order for when the time is right to welcome and grow a baby."

Explanation

After the story, which may be at the same time or later you can provide a more detailed explanation:

"Menstruation is a natural process that prepares the body for a potential pregnancy and occurs in four phases: shedding the old uterine lining during the period, preparing a new egg and thickening the uterine lining in the follicular phase, releasing an egg during ovulation, and in the luteal phase, the body maintains the uterine lining in case of pregnancy. If fertilisation doesn't occur, hormone levels drop, signalling the body to shed the lining and start a new cycle.

We can also talk about ways to manage the bleeding during your menstrual phase, and I can show you what I use—things you've already seen in my bag and bathroom. This cycle is a sign of a healthy, functioning reproductive system, our bodies are incredible!"

Adapt, Personalise and Community Support

Feel free to adapt this story and explanation to suit your needs and what feels right for you, but I hope this gives you a little idea of how you can make this a positive learning experience. By presenting periods in a positive light and emphasising the body's intelligence and natural processes, we can help normalise menstruation and reduce the stigma and negativity often associated with it.

There are many beautiful ways to find community support, Charlotte Pointeaux runs First Moon Circles, an empowering menstrual education program for girls aged 9-12. These circles provide a nurturing space where girls can learn about periods and puberty in a positive, supportive environment.

I also encourage you to check out Amanda Trieger's empowering puberty workshops and retreats. Designed for mothers, healers, and practitioners, these sessions guide young girls through menarche with wisdom and community support. Amanda provides practical tools to empower girls, ensuring their journey into womanhood is celebrated, with over two decades of experience in women's health.

You can find additional resources and ways to connect with these amazing programs in the resource section.

Chapter 6
Origins of Seed Cycling

Seed cycling, also known as seed rotation or menstrual seeds, is widely embraced in natural health communities and recognised in naturopathic and functional medicine circles.

I am particularly driven to investigate the historical roots of the individual seeds and the beginnings of the seed cycling practice. Additionally, the compelling stories I've encountered inspire my interest in understanding its evolution and significance even further.

Over the years, I have come to love and appreciate how eager people are to share their seed cycling experiences with me. I'd love to share a few that have particularly stuck in my mind.

One woman told me how she was introduced to seed cycling over a decade ago by an acupuncturist who swore by its efficacy for hormonal balance. She followed the acupuncturist's advice and noticed significant improvements in her menstrual cycle and PMS symptoms.

Another compelling story came from a woman whose naturopath, practicing ancient healing methods recommended seed cycling to support her fertility. Remarkably, she conceived a few months after starting the practice and credits seed cycling for her successful pregnancy.

One more memorable story is from a woman who has been seed cycling for over 20 years. She credits the nutrients in the seeds for her easy menopause transition, attributing her smooth experience to the consistent support seed cycling provided her hormones over the years.

These stories resonate deeply with me, illustrating the diverse ways in which seed cycling has been shared and embraced. They highlight the personal journeys and profound impacts this practice can have. While I regret not documenting these stories more thoroughly and noting the names of the practitioners, these experiences underscore the importance of exploring the rich history and potential benefits of seed cycling.

The History of Seeds

Seeds have played a profound role in diverse cultures across history, valued for their nutritional benefits and therapeutic qualities. Dating back millennia, civilisations have revered specific seeds for their capacity to enhance bodily equilibrium and overall vitality.

Ancient Ayurvedic texts and Chinese medical literature provide insight into the historical significance of seeds in traditional healing practices. The seeds of plants are endowed with various properties and are used for their medicinal benefits. Pumpkin seeds are nourishing and help in maintaining digestive health. Sesame seeds are considered to be beneficial for hormonal balance and reproductive health. They are often used in herbal formulations to support women's health.

Historical references demonstrate the enduring legacy of seed-based remedies in ancient healing traditions and provide a foundation for the modern practice of seed cycling as a natural approach to hormonal balance and overall well-being.

While seed cycling may not be explicitly mentioned in these texts, the use of seeds to support hormones aligns with the principles of these ancient practices.

Seeds used in Ayurveda

In Ayurveda, the ancient healing system of India, seeds have been valued for their therapeutic effects on the body and mind. Ayurvedic texts such as the "Charaka Samhita" and the "Sushruta Samhita" describe the medicinal properties of seeds like pumpkin and sunflower, highlighting their role in promoting health.

Pumpkin seeds, known as "Kushmanda" in Sanskrit, were prized for their nourishing properties and were believed to support digestive health and vitality. Sunflower seeds, referred to as "Suryabhakta," were esteemed for their ability to balance the doshas (bioenergetic forces) within the body and enhance energy levels.

There are also details of the use of seeds in fertility treatments and reproductive health support. Seeds like sesame, flax, and pumpkin are incorporated into Ayurvedic formulations to balance the doshas (energetic forces) and promote fertility.

Traditional Chinese Medicine (TCM) Seeds

In ancient China, seeds held a prominent role in promoting health, deeply rooted in Traditional Chinese Medicine (TCM) practices. Certain seeds were revered for their unique capacity to enhance bodily balance and vitality. For instance, flaxseeds were prized for their rich Omega-3 fatty acids, traditionally believed to bolster heart health and cognitive function. Similarly, sesame seeds were highly esteemed within TCM for their nourishing attributes and potential to support hormonal equilibrium.

TCM Seeds for Fertility and Reproduction

The concept of using seeds to generate "seeds" underscores the holistic approach of TCM for fertility support. By harnessing the innate potential of seeds, TCM practitioners aim to cultivate vitality and balance within the body, thereby enhancing fertility outcomes.

Drawing from centuries of TCM wisdom, we can recognise the profound impact that medicinal seeds can have on reproductive health. The use of seeds for fertility and reproductive health extends beyond traditional TCM and is found in various natural healing practices worldwide. The origins of seed-based therapies can be traced back to ancient civilisations, where seeds were revered for their medicinal properties and symbolic significance.

In the realm of Chinese herbology, seeds play a crucial role in supporting fertility and reproductive health. Herbal formulas crafted from seeds are highly valued for their ability to nourish and invigorate the body, particularly in cases of diminished ovarian reserve or low sperm count.

Similarly, in traditional European herbalism, seeds have been valued for their nutritive and medicinal properties. Herbalists throughout history have recognised the role of seeds in supporting reproductive health and have formulated remedies using seeds such as chia, hemp, and sunflower to address fertility issues and hormonal imbalances.

Evolution of Seed Cycling as a Natural Remedy for Hormone Balance

Seed cycling, as we know it today has become a phenomenon gaining traction with the proliferation of social media, marking its initial appearance on the internet during the late 20th century.

Discussions about seed cycling began to emerge in alternative health forums, wellness blogs, and social media platforms. Websites dedicated to natural remedies, holistic health practices, and women's wellness may have been among the earliest sources to mention seed cycling in the modern world.

As the collective wisdom grew, so did the understanding of seed cycling's potential benefits. Described as menstrual biohacking, it emerged as a holistic approach to addressing a myriad of menstrual cycle issues, ranging from PMS symptoms and hormonal acne breakouts to supporting fertility and easing the transition through menopause.

While its precise origins are not definitively documented, the practice has historical roots in traditional healing practices. New science and research as well as anecdotal evidence and personal testimonies continue to fuel its popularity among individuals, practitioners and doctors seeking natural alternatives for hormone balance. As our understanding of the intricate interplay between diet, lifestyle, and hormonal health deepens, seed cycling stands as a testament to the enduring appeal of holistic approaches to wellness.

History of the Four Key Seeds for Seed Cycling

Let us delve into the rich history of the four key seeds used in seed cycling: flaxseeds, pumpkin seeds, sesame seeds, and sunflower seeds. Exploring the historical roots and traditional uses of these seeds provides valuable insights and a deeper appreciation for their long-standing significance in various cultures. By understanding their historical context, we can better appreciate the enduring value and applications of these seeds in promoting health and food as medicine.

History of Flaxseeds

Flaxseeds have been cultivated for thousands of years and have their origins in ancient Mesopotamia (modern-day Iraq and Iran). They were one of the first crops to be domesticated by humans, with evidence of their use dating back to at least 5,000 BCE. From Mesopotamia, flax cultivation spread to other regions of the world, including Egypt, Greece, and eventually Europe and North America.

Historically, flaxseeds have been used for a variety of purposes:

Food: Flaxseeds have long been valued as a nutritious food source. In ancient times, they were often consumed in various forms, including as a ground powder or pressed into oils. Flaxseed oil was particularly prized for its culinary and medicinal properties.

> **Textiles**: Flax fibres, derived from the stalks of the flax plant, were used to make linen textiles. Linen fabric was highly valued in ancient civilisations for its durability, breathability, and versatility. Flax cultivation was integral to the textile industry in regions where it was grown.

> **Medicine**: Flaxseeds were also used for medicinal purposes in ancient cultures. They were believed to have various health benefits, including promoting digestion, relieving constipation, and soothing inflammation. Flaxseed poultices were sometimes applied topically to treat wounds and skin conditions.

Religious and Cultural Practices: Flaxseeds had symbolic significance in many cultures. In ancient Egypt, for example, flax was associated with the goddess Isis and was used in religious ceremonies and rituals. They were also a common motif in art and architecture, representing concepts such as fertility, regeneration, and purity.

History of Pumpkin Seeds

Pumpkin seeds have a rich history and origins dating back thousands of years:

Ancient Civilisations: Pumpkin seeds were a staple food in the diet of indigenous peoples in the Americas, particularly in regions where pumpkins and squash were cultivated. Archaeological evidence suggests that pumpkin seeds were consumed by Native American tribes as early as 7000 BCE.

Culinary Uses: Indigenous cultures in the Americas used pumpkin seeds in various culinary preparations. They were often roasted, ground into meal or flour, or used as a thickening agent in soups and stews. Pumpkin seeds were valued for their nutritional content and versatility in cooking.

Medicinal Purposes: In addition to being a dietary staple, pumpkin seeds were also used for medicinal purposes by indigenous peoples. They were believed to have various health benefits, including supporting digestion, promoting urinary tract health, and alleviating intestinal parasites.

Cultural Significance: Pumpkin seeds held cultural significance for many indigenous tribes in the Americas. They were used in religious ceremonies, rituals, and celebrations, symbolising abundance, fertility, and sustenance. Pumpkin seeds were often included as offerings in traditional ceremonies and feasts.

European Introduction: Pumpkin seeds were introduced to Europe by explorers and settlers returning from the Americas. They became popular in European cuisine, where they were used in both sweet and savory dishes. Pumpkin seeds were also valued for their nutritional benefits and were incorporated into traditional herbal remedies.

History of Sesame Seeds

Originating in Africa and India, sesame seeds have been cultivated since ancient times for their nutritional value and medicinal properties. Historical evidence suggests that sesame seeds were used as early as 3000 BCE in these regions.

> **Culinary Uses**: Sesame seeds were incorporated into culinary dishes across different cultures, adding a nutty flavour and a nutritional boost to a wide range of foods. They were used to make oils, pastes, and powders, enhancing both sweet and savory dishes.
>
> **Medicinal Purposes**: In addition to their culinary applications, sesame seeds were believed to have various healing properties. They were used to make oils and pastes thought to reduce inflammation, support digestion, and improve skin health.
>
> **Cultural Significance**: Sesame seeds held cultural significance in many ancient societies. They were often included in rituals and traditional medicine practices, symbolising health and prosperity. The seeds were considered a valuable trade commodity due to their versatile uses and benefits.
>
> **Spread to Other Regions**: As trade routes expanded, sesame seeds were introduced to various parts of the world. They became popular in Middle Eastern, Mediterranean, and Asian cuisines, continuing to be valued for their nutritional benefits and versatility in cooking and medicine.

History of Sunflower Seeds

Sunflower seeds have a fascinating history that dates back thousands of years. Originating in North and Central America, sunflowers were initially cultivated by indigenous peoples, particularly in regions that are now part of Mexico and the southwestern United States. These ancient civilisations not only appreciated the sunflower's beauty but also recognised its nutritional value and versatility.

Indigenous Cultures: The sunflower plant played a significant role in indigenous cultures, serving as a source of food, medicine, and dye. The seeds were harvested and consumed as a nutrient-rich food source, providing essential fats, protein, and micronutrients.

European Encounter: European explorers encountered sunflowers during their travels to the Americas in the 16th century. They brought sunflower seeds back to Europe, where the plant gained popularity as a decorative flower and a valuable oilseed crop.

Culinary and Industrial Uses: Sunflower oil, extracted from the seeds, became a staple ingredient in European cuisine and was also used for various industrial purposes.

Russian Cultivation: In the 18th century, Russian farmers began cultivating sunflowers on a larger scale for their oil-rich seeds. The practice spread rapidly across Russia and eventually to other parts of Europe and Asia.

Widespread Cultivation: By the 19th century, sunflower cultivation had become widespread, particularly in Russia, Ukraine, and other regions with favourable growing conditions, solidifying the sunflower's status as an important agricultural crop.

Modern Day Seed Oils

Sunflower oil quickly gained popularity in European cuisine for its light flavour and high smoke point, making it suitable for frying, baking, and salad dressings. Its widespread use in cooking contributed to its status as a staple ingredient in European households.

However, as industrialisation and chemical processes advanced, the production of sunflower seed oil underwent significant changes. Modern methods of extraction often involve the use of high heat, chemical solvents, and refining processes, which can degrade the oil's nutritional quality and introduce harmful substances.

Processed sunflower seed oil may contain high levels of unhealthy trans fats, oxidation byproducts, and residues from chemical solvents used during extraction. Additionally, refined sunflower oil may lack the beneficial nutrients found in cold-pressed or unrefined oils.

As a result, health experts caution against the consumption of highly processed sunflower seed oil.

Doctors and Hormone Experts on Seed Cycling

Naturopathic doctors and holistic practitioners often incorporate seed cycling into treatment protocols for conditions such as irregular menstruation, PMS, and hormonal imbalances. Many are also calling for more research to fully understand the efficacy of seed cycling.

Dr. Jolene Brighten a prominent naturopathic physician and women's health expert, has been instrumental in bringing seed cycling to the forefront of holistic wellness practices.

> "Seed cycling has long been used to support women's hormones by supplying them with the nutrients they need at specific phases of their cycle. I recommend seed cycling for hormone balance in both my clinic and book, Beyond the Pill, because it is an effective and gentle way to support women's hormones. Seed cycling provides the specific nutrients to help build your hormones.
>
> I recommend seed cycling at any stage in a woman's life and find it especially helpful for women coming off of birth control or struggling with post-birth control syndrome symptoms like acne, irregular periods, or new onset of PMS. To use seed cycling you need to know a few things.
>
> You'll be tracking your menstrual cycle and changing your seeds to match the phase you are in. Day one is the first day you experience your period (there is a flow). That will be the day

you begin the follicular phase seeds, and you'll continue through ovulation or day 14." **– Dr Jolene Brighten, Functional Medicine Naturopathic Physician**

Alisa Vitti, a Functional Nutritionist and author of the famous book "In the Flow," has also played a significant role in popularising seed cycling as a tool for hormonal balance. In her book, Vitti outlines the science behind seed cycling and provides practical guidance for incorporating it into one's daily routine.

"Try seed cycling, some women have experienced reduction in hormonal symptoms by consuming certain seeds as part of their cyclical routine." - **Alisa Vitti, In The Flow.**

"Seed cycling is one significant way to boost your hormonal health by taking advantage of certain seeds' natural hormonal balancing, antioxidant, and anti-inflammatory properties. In addition to a balanced diet, seed cycling can completely change the way you relate to your hormones." **Dr Mark Hyman**

Australian Nutritionist's Steph Lowe and Tris Alexandra Jarvis share:

"Seed cycling is one of my favourite nutritional strategies for balanced hormones, healthy periods, regular ovulation, clear skin and stable moods. I recommend The Seed Cycle™ to all of my clients and online community." **Steph Lowe- The Natural Nutritionist**

"Seed cycling is a great nutritional practice that not only helps women gain a deeper connection to their menstrual cycle rhythm, but also supports their body as part of a natural and nutritional approach to hormone health that is gentle and effective.

The seeds provide many of the nutrients the body needs to support hormone production and balance through the different phases of our menstrual cycle, and I've witnessed great improvements in irregular cycles, PCOS symptoms, skin breakouts, and hormonal symptoms post coming off hormonal birth control using seed cycling with my clients." **- Tris**

Alexandra Jarvis, Clinical Nutritionist, BHSc & Natural Fertility/Menstrual Cycle Educator

Amanda Trieger, Lead Naturopath at Naturopathic Womancraft Clinic and Trainer for Health Professionals shares:

> "As a naturopath, I've witnessed how this practice nurtures hormonal balance by aligning nutrition with a woman's menstrual phases. Seed cycling works to gently support the body's natural rhythm, providing estrogen-enhancing seeds like flax and pumpkin during the follicular phase and progesterone-supporting seeds like sesame and sunflower in the luteal phase.
>
> It's a simple yet profound practice that uses nature's gifts to harmonize the intricate dance of hormones. I utlise it for women in all phases of life from puberty, cyclical years and the menstrual menopause transition." – **Amanda Trieger, (B.Nat, NHAA, SCU, SW Glad, EL) Lead Naturopath at Naturopathic Womancraft Clinic, Trainer for Health Professionals, Vaginal Microbiome Specialist, Pre & Post-partum Doula**

In the beauty industry, leaders like Kim Le Sambolic emphasize the transformative power of seed cycling for skin health. As she states,

> "We highly recommend seed cycling to support our client skin transformation journeys. The seeds work magic by boosting the body's nutrient reserves, helping to rebuild skin health from within. Our clients find it easy and delicious to add to any meal or drink. Studies confirm these nutrient-rich seeds strengthen the skin's barrier and maintain a healthy balance with only positive effects." – **Kim Le Sambolic CEO/Dermal Clinician, Skin Wellness Academy**

Chapter 7
Seed Cycling Nutrients, Science and Research

In this chapter, join me as I celebrate and explore the nutritional richness and therapeutic properties of the seeds used in seed cycling. I will delve into the current scientific validation and research on seed cycling as a practice, accompanied by case studies from The Seed Cycle™.

I have recently seen some scepticism on social media, dismissing seed cycling as a 'trend' and one dietitian calling it 'bullshit'. It's understandable why some may be sceptical about seed cycling, especially when it hasn't been widely studied or taught in formal education, like in dietetics. Without an abundance of peer-reviewed research or hundreds of scientific papers to back it up, seed cycling can easily be dismissed as a "trend" or seen as too simplistic of a solution for something as complex as hormone balance. For those trained to rely on hard data and clinical studies only, it might seem unconvincing.

Interestingly, I have personally only been met with positivity and curiosity when introducing seed cycling both in person and online. I have connected with hundreds of practitioners and experts, as well as the thousands of customers who have seed cycled with my company, attesting to its benefits as a functional food, reducing hormone imbalance symptoms.

Let's begin by examining the unique qualities and abundant nutrients found in the four key seeds used in seed cycling. The true benefits of this practice lie in the extraordinary nutrients these humble seeds provide.

As I delve into the science and research behind seed cycling, it's important to acknowledge the historical context of women's health research. For many years, women were often excluded from clinical trials, creating a significant gap in our understanding of their health issues. It wasn't until the late 20th century that this began to change, particularly with the passage of the National Institutes of Health (NIH) Revitalization Act of 1993, which mandated the inclusion of women and minorities in NIH-funded research. This legislation recognised the importance of understanding how medical treatments affect different genders. Before this shift, the lack of representation in studies relied heavily on male-centric data, which frequently overlooked the unique physiological and hormonal differences in women.

Consequently, health guidelines and treatment protocols were often less effective or even harmful to women. Ongoing research underscores the need for gender-specific studies to ensure that women's health needs are adequately addressed, ultimately improving overall health outcomes.

Flaxseeds

Flaxseed and linseed are terms often used interchangeably, but there can be slight differences depending on regional conventions and specific varieties. However, in general, flaxseed and linseed refer to the same seed, obtained from the flax plant, *Linum usitatissimum*.

Given their similar nutritional profiles and uses, flaxseeds and linseeds can both be used for seed cycling without any impact on the overall effectiveness of the practice.

However, it's important to note that flaxseed meal, often found in supermarkets, isn't the same as whole ground flaxseeds. Ground flaxseed retains the full spectrum of nutrients, including fibre, lignans, and omega-3 fatty acids, all of which contribute to hormone balance.

Flaxseed meal, on the other hand, is often made from the byproduct left after the oil has been extracted, meaning it can lack some of these key nutrients, especially the essential fats.

The Research and Studies on Flaxseed Nutrients

Flaxseeds have gained attention for their potential to alleviate menstrual problems. Studies suggest they can lengthen the luteal phase, improve ovulation, and reduce premenstrual symptoms like breast pain and cramping. This is largely due to lignans, a compound abundantly found in flaxseeds.

Flaxseeds also offer diverse health benefits beyond hormone regulation. Their lignans and Omega-3 fatty acids reduce inflammation and support regular bowel movements.

Rich in antioxidants like lignans and polyphenols, flaxseeds protect against oxidative stress, lowering the risk of chronic diseases such as heart disease and cancer. They also provide plant-based protein crucial for tissue repair and growth, along with essential vitamins (B1, magnesium, phosphorus, selenium) supporting energy metabolism, bone health, and immune function.

Research indicates that incorporating flaxseeds into the diet improves cardiovascular health by lowering blood pressure and cholesterol levels, again thanks to their Omega-3 fatty acids, fibre, and lignans.

Phytoestrogens in Flaxseeds

This section delves into some technical aspects, my hope is that you come to appreciate the remarkable role flaxseeds play in supporting hormone health. These small yet powerful seeds are rich in lignans, a specific type of phytoestrogen renowned for their unique ability to influence hormone levels effectively.

Lignans, predominantly found in flaxseeds, possess both estrogenic and anti-estrogenic properties. This dual capability allows them to modulate hormone activity.

Incredibly, these compounds have molecular structures akin to endogenous estradiol, allowing them to bind to estrogen receptors in the body. These receptors, classified into alpha and beta types, serve distinct roles: alpha receptors promote cell proliferation (the process of cells growing and dividing) while beta receptors facilitate cell apoptosis (the process of programmed cell death that helps eliminate unhealthy cells).

Once phytoestrogens bind to these receptors, they migrate from the cytoplasm to the cell nucleus, influencing gene expression through DNA transcription processes. This means they have a dual role in supporting and helping regulate healthy estrogen levels.

Early research raised concerns that flaxseeds might negatively impact estrogen by increasing sex hormone-binding globulin (SHBG) protein concentration. However, more recent studies have challenged and disproven this view, showing that flaxseeds help modulate estrogen levels and aid in metabolised estrogen excretion, promoting hormonal balance.

Phytoestrogens are metabolised in the gut, where intestinal bacteria break them down before they are absorbed and processed in the liver. Afterward, these compounds circulate in the bloodstream until they are excreted in the urine. Due to their structural similarity to natural estrogen, phytoestrogens can influence estrogen-regulated processes, such as inhibiting the aromatase enzyme (which converts androgens into estrogens) and affecting the regulation of SHBG.

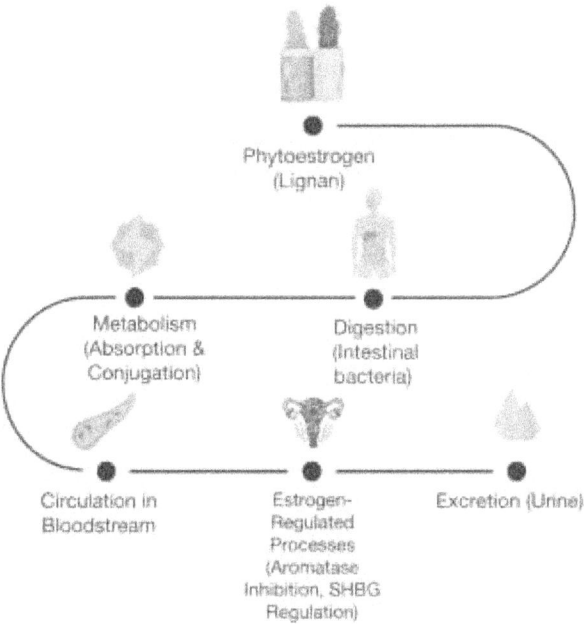

Figure 2. The Seed Cycle™ Estrogen Pathway

*This diagram illustrates the journey of phytoestrogens from ingestion through digestion and metabolism, circulation in the bloodstream, and eventual excretion. Along the way, phytoestrogens influence estrogen-regulated processes such as aromatase inhibition and sex hormone-binding globulin regulation due to their structural similarity to endogenous estrogen.

Phytoestrogens for Weight Management

Phytoestrogens also play a role in weight management, particularly due to lignans' ability to enhance fat-free mass, reduce fat accumulation, and decrease serum leptin levels (leptin is a hormone involved in regulating appetite and energy balance). Research suggests that flaxseed lignans contribute to significant reductions in visceral fat and serum leptin concentrations.

Animal studies further indicate that lignans can suppress appetite and induce apoptosis in adipocytes (fat cells), which may aid in weight reduction.

Phytoestrogens Supporting Regular Menstrual Cycles

Notably, lignans are associated with a longer luteal phase and reduced anovulatory cycles, enhancing the likelihood of regular ovulation. They can also improve the progesterone to estrogen ratio during the luteal phase and reduce excess estrogen levels, beneficial for those with irregular periods or low progesterone.

Targeted Nutrient Dosages from Flaxseeds

Here is a breakdown of the doses reported in studies for nutrients found in flaxseeds, as they relate to hormone health and specific conditions:

Lignans (Phytoestrogens):

> **Study**: Daily doses of 25-50 grams of flax seeds are effective for hormone balance, managing menopause symptoms, and reducing PMS.
>
> **Sources**: Studies on flax lignans and hormone modulation recommend 25 grams/day for significant estrogen balancing effects, particularly in postmenopausal women.

Omega-3 Fatty Acids:

> **Study**: The optimal intake of alpha-linolenic acid (ALA, a type of Omega-3) from flaxseeds is 1.1-1.6 grams/day for adult women.
>
> **Sources**: Research supports that consuming 1 tablespoon of ground flaxseeds daily can meet the ALA needs of adult women, promoting cardiovascular and overall health.

Seed Cycling:

> Applying 1 tablespoon of ground flaxseed as part of your seed cycling practice during the follicular phase can help you meet the daily recommended intake of lignans and omega-3 fatty acids.

Pumpkin Seeds

The botanical name for the pumpkin seed plant is *Cucurbita pepo*. Pumpkin seeds are nutrient-rich seeds harvested from pumpkins, a member of the squash family.

While the terms "pumpkin seeds" and "pepitas" are often used interchangeably, there are subtle differences between the two. Pumpkin seeds refer to the entire seed, including the outer shell, while pepitas specifically denote the seed without the outer hull. Pepitas have a smaller, greener appearance compared to pumpkin seeds, which are larger and often encased in a white shell. Despite these variances, both pumpkin seeds and pepitas offer numerous health benefits and both can be used for seed cycling.

The Research and Studies on Pumpkin Seeds Nutrients

Pumpkin seeds have been the subject of numerous studies due to their nutrient density, which plays a significant role in supporting women's hormonal health.

Pumpkin seeds are particularly high in zinc, a crucial mineral for hormone production. Research indicates that zinc is essential to produce progesterone, a hormone that plays a key role in the menstrual cycle and pregnancy. Zinc stimulates the release of Follicle Stimulating Hormone (FSH), which is necessary for ovulation and, consequently, the production of progesterone. Studies have shown that adequate zinc levels are associated with better ovulation and overall reproductive health, making it vital for women trying to conceive or maintain a healthy menstrual cycle.

Pumpkin seeds are also a rich source of magnesium, another mineral vital for women's health. Magnesium plays a critical role in reducing menstrual pain and supporting a healthy stress response. Stress is known to interfere with ovulation by disrupting the balance of hormones, particularly cortisol. By promoting relaxation and reducing stress, magnesium helps ensure that progesterone levels remain balanced.

In addition to zinc and magnesium, pumpkin seeds contain Omega-3 fatty acids, including beta-sitosterol. These fatty acids are beneficial for controlling insulin levels and reducing inflammation, both of which are important for managing conditions like PCOS. Omega-3s have been shown in studies to reduce elevated androgen levels, by lowering these androgens, Omega-3s from pumpkin seeds help support a more balanced hormonal environment.

Targeted Nutrient Dosages from Pumpkin Seeds

Here is a breakdown of the doses reported in studies for nutrients found in pumpkin seeds, as they relate to hormone health and specific conditions:

Zinc

>**Study**: Research has shown that doses of 15-30 mg/day of zinc are effective in regulating hormone levels, better ovulation, and supporting progesterone production in women.
>
>**Sources**: Most studies recommend around 1-2 tablespoons of pumpkin seeds daily to meet part of the zinc needs.

Magnesium

>**Study**: In clinical trials, 200-400 mg/day of magnesium has been shown to alleviate menstrual cramps, promote better sleep, and improve stress response during the luteal phase.
>
>**Sources**: ¼ cup (28 grams) of pumpkin seeds provides approximately 150 mg of magnesium, which contributes significantly toward daily intake.

Seed Cycling:

>Adding 1 tablespoon of ground pumpkin seeds as part of your seed cycling process during the follicular phase can help you obtain essential nutrients, including magnesium, zinc, and omega-6 fatty acids.

Sunflower Seeds

The botanical name for the sunflower seed plant is *Helianthus annuus*. Sunflower seeds are nutrient-dense seeds harvested from sunflowers, which belong to the Asteraceae family.

Sunflower seeds are packed with essential nutrients. They are an excellent source of healthy fats, primarily polyunsaturated and monounsaturated fats, which are beneficial for heart health.

The Research and Studies on Sunflower Seeds

Sunflower seeds offer significant benefits for women's hormonal health due to their rich nutrient profile. Selenium in sunflower seeds, an essential mineral that the body requires in small amounts, supports liver function, aiding the removal of excess estrogen from the body and contributing to hormonal balance.

Additionally, sunflower seeds are a good source of Vitamin E, which provides antioxidant protection and supports progesterone production.

Recent research highlights the combined effects of selenium and Vitamin E in positively impacting ovarian reserves and fertility, making them key nutrients for women's reproductive health.

Moreover, the essential fatty acids (EFAs) in sunflower seeds can convert to gamma-linolenic acid (GLA), which helps alleviate pre-menstrual breast tenderness. During the luteal phase of the menstrual cycle, the body is better able to utilise EFAs, emphasising their importance for hormonal regulation.

Together, the nutrients in sunflower seeds—particularly selenium and Vitamin E—work to support liver function, regulate estrogen, boost progesterone production, and enhance thyroid health, all of which contribute to a balanced hormonal system.

Targeted Nutrient Dosages from Sunflower Seeds

Here is a breakdown of the doses reported in studies for nutrients found in sunflower seeds, as they relate to hormone health and specific conditions:

Selenium

> **Study**: Selenium doses of 55-200 mcg/day are commonly recommended for supporting liver function, estrogen detoxification, and thyroid health.

Sources: 28 grams of sunflower seeds provides about 20-25 mcg of selenium, meaning multiple servings or combined sources are often needed to meet daily selenium needs.

Vitamin E

Study: The typical recommended dose of Vitamin E for reducing PMS and supporting fertility is 15-30 mg/day.

Sources: 28 grams of sunflower seeds contains 7.4 mg of Vitamin E, meaning 53 grams can meet or exceed daily recommendations.

Seed Cycling:

Adding 1 tablespoon of ground sunflower seeds as part of your seed cycling process during the luteal phase can help you obtain vital nutrients such as vitamin E, selenium, and magnesium.

Sesame Seeds

Sesame seeds, derived from the *Sesamum indicum* plant, have a rich history spanning centuries. These tiny seeds, packed with nutrients and flavour, have been a staple in cuisines around the world for millennia.

The Research and Studies on Sesame Seeds

Sesame seeds are not only rich in zinc and lignans but also contain significant amounts of calcium and vitamin B6, which play essential roles in women's hormonal health. Calcium is crucial for maintaining muscle and nerve function, and its presence in sesame seeds has been linked to reducing PMS symptoms such as cramps, mood swings, and fatigue. Additionally, vitamin B6 aids in mood regulation, helping to alleviate symptoms of depression and anxiety associated with PMS.

A study published in the *Reproductive Health Journal* in 2021 highlights the role of sesame lignans in enhancing estrogen metabolism and improving Perimenopause function, showing promise for boosting fertility in women with low estrogen levels. This makes sesame seeds particularly useful for those struggling with fertility issues related to hormonal imbalances.

Further supporting menstrual health, a 2020 study from the *Journal of Women's Health* found that the anti-inflammatory properties of sesame seed oil help ease menstrual cramps and alleviate PMS symptoms by improving circulation and promoting hormonal balance. This combination of calcium, vitamin B6, and anti-inflammatory compounds in sesame seeds offers a comprehensive approach to managing menstrual discomfort and supporting fertility.

Targeted Nutrient Dosages from Sesame Seeds

Here is a breakdown of the doses reported in studies for nutrients found in sesame seeds, as they relate to hormone health and specific conditions:

Lignans

> **Study**: Research on sesame seeds suggests that 50-100 mg/day of lignans can help in regulating estrogen levels and reducing androgen-related symptoms like acne.
>
> **Sources**: 1 tablespoon of sesame seeds contains about 30 mg of lignans, meaning a few tablespoons daily could support hormonal health.

Calcium

> **Study**: Studies indicate that calcium intake in the range of 500-1000 mg/day is beneficial for reducing PMS symptoms and supporting overall reproductive health.
>
> **Sources:** Sesame seeds contribute around 90 mg of calcium per tablespoon, which can help meet this need.

Seed Cycling:

> Adding tablespoon of ground sesame seeds into your seed cycling routine during the luteal phase can help you achieve your daily intake of essential nutrients such as calcium, magnesium, and lignans.

When examining specific seed dosages based on research, it becomes clear that the seed cycling recommended doses align well with recommendations for nutrients like zinc, magnesium, lignans, and essential fatty acids. By incorporating these seeds in daily portions of 1-2 tablespoons each, many individuals can achieve the recommended doses of these key nutrients to support hormone health naturally.

The Seed Cycling Connection: Aligning Hormonal Forces

Now that we have explored the nutrients and research for seed cycling seeds and how they work in isolation let's look at how they work together. The combined nutritional benefits of these seeds play a crucial role in supporting hormone balance and overall health.

Fibre and Gut Health

Fibre plays a crucial role in seed cycling, promoting both digestive and hormonal health. Seeds, with their high fibre content (around 10%), support regular bowel movements and help the body eliminate excess estrogen, preventing estrogen dominance.

The estrobolome, a collection of gut bacteria, is responsible for metabolising and regulating estrogen levels. When the estrobolome is healthy and supported by a fibre-rich diet, it efficiently processes estrogen, reducing the risk of hormonal imbalances like bloating and irregular periods. Fibre from seeds nourishes beneficial gut bacteria, enhancing the estrobolome's function and promoting balanced hormone levels.

Magnesium

Essential for estrogen breakdown, gut function, and mood regulation, magnesium is found in flax, pumpkin, sesame, and sunflower seeds, helping alleviate period pain and support muscle health.

Iron

Crucial for energy and nervous system health, iron from pumpkin and sesame seeds replenishes stores lost during menstruation, ensuring optimal bodily function.

Manganese

A potent antioxidant essential for bone and thyroid health, manganese is particularly abundant in pumpkin seeds.

Vitamin E

Present in pumpkin and sunflower seeds, Vitamin E boosts progesterone levels and corrects estrogen-progesterone imbalances.

Selenium

Sunflower seeds are rich in selenium, a vital nutrient for cognitive and heart health, while sesame seeds also provide this antioxidant.

Calcium

Sesame seeds contribute to calcium intake, crucial for bone and muscle function, as well as hormone release, helping reduce period pain.

Healthy Fats

Seeds contain heart-healthy polyunsaturated and monounsaturated fats, including Omega-3s, promoting satiety and balanced blood sugar levels.

Phytosterols

These plant compounds have a structure like cholesterol and may help lower cholesterol levels in the blood. Pumpkin seeds, used in seed cycling, are a good source of phytosterols. They also have anti-inflammatory and immune-modulating effects.

Polyphenols

Found in all four seed cycling seeds, act as antioxidants, aiding in hormonal balance, cardiovascular health, and cognitive function for women. They're crucial for overall well-being, especially during menstruation, menopause, and reproductive health stages.

The Seed Cycle™ Nutritional Benefits Summarised

The Seed Cycle™ Phase 1 (Organic Flaxseeds and Pumpkin Seeds, 1 serving)

> More than 100% of the recommended daily intake for Omega-3 (ALA)
>
> 25% of daily magnesium
>
> 14% of daily manganese
>
> 12.5% of daily zinc
>
> 7% of daily iron
>
> 6% of daily selenium

The Seed Cycle™ Phase 2 (Organic Sunflower Seeds and Sesame Seeds, 1 serving)

> 47% of daily Vitamin E
>
> 20% of daily magnesium
>
> 10% of daily calcium
>
> 9.5% of daily iron
>
> 6% of daily selenium
>
> 6% of daily zinc

The Scientific Validation of Seed Cycling

There is a growing body of research that demonstrate the benefits of seed cycling for women's hormone health and specific health conditions. There has been research conducted on seed cycling as a practice including a promising review published in January 2021 on seed cycling for PCOS and more recently in June 2023 a study on the effectiveness of combined seeds (pumpkin, sunflower, sesame, flaxseed) as adjacent therapy to treat polycystic ovary syndrome in females.

In Chapter 11, we delve deeper into the seed cycling PCOS study as it sheds light on the potential benefits of seed cycling as a dietary intervention for managing PCOS symptoms.

A review titled "Advantages of Seed Cycling Diet in Menstrual Dysfunctions: A Review Based Explanation," published in February 2023, underscores the importance of further investigation into the efficacy of seed cycling as a therapeutic approach for addressing various menstrual dysfunctions. The review suggests that seed cycling has promising potential as a diet-based therapy, but more research is required to establish its evidence-based, dose-dependent effectiveness in improving female menstrual health.

It is great that we have this research available to us, shedding light on the potential benefits of seed cycling for women's health. However, considering the vast importance of women's health and the potential impact of interventions like seed cycling, it's clear that further research is necessary. Investing in additional studies in this area could lead to invaluable insights and advancements in supporting women's health.

Seed Cycling Case Studies

As a company, The Seed Cycle™ collaborates closely with naturopaths and nutritionists to gather data on the effectiveness of seed cycling as a natural approach to hormonal balance. These practitioners work with clients of diverse backgrounds, addressing various health concerns, ages, lifestyles, and medical histories.

In each case study, the practitioner provides a brief overview of the client's health concerns, including any relevant details about their age, lifestyle, and medical history. Seed cycling is introduced as part of the client's health regimen over a period of three months, allowing ample time to observe changes and adjustments along the way.

Throughout the case study, practitioners document any changes in menstrual regularity, hormone balance, fertility indicators, mood, energy levels, and physical signs or symptoms of hormonal imbalance. They may also include data from hormonal testing, such as bloodwork, to provide a comprehensive assessment of the client's progress.

In addition to seed cycling, practitioners may integrate additional recommendations, lifestyle changes, or therapies to enhance the client's results. These complementary approaches may include dietary modifications, stress management techniques, herbal supplements, or other supportive therapies tailored to the client's individual needs.

Upon completion of the case study, practitioners summarise the overall outcomes and impact of seed cycling on the client's health and well-being. Importantly, no incentives are provided to practitioners for completing these case studies, ensuring the integrity and objectivity of the data gathered.

Naturopath Case Study 1 – Hormonal Acne Post Pill

Client Background:	The client is a 30-year-old female with a history of using the contraceptive pill and intermittently taking the medication Roaccutane since the age of 16 to manage hormonal acne. She has been experiencing hormonal headaches severe enough to incapacitate her for several days at a time, accompanied by symptoms such as nausea and an inability to eat or perform regular activities.
Description:	A few months ago, after consulting with her GP, the client decided to discontinue the use of the contraceptive pill, suspecting that it may have been exacerbating her headaches. Following the discontinuation of the pill, she noticed breakouts on her skin, particularly around her chin. Additionally, her menstrual period has not returned, raising concerns about her hormonal health.
Progress and Changes:	Over the 4-month period of seed cycling use, the client noticed significant improvement in her skin within the first month. New breakouts ceased to occur, and existing breakouts were healing. Shortly after initiating seed cycling, the client experienced her first menstrual period since discontinuing the contraceptive pill. Although the initial period was light and short (lasting only 2 days), the return of menstruation indicated progress in regulating her hormonal balance and menstrual cycle. During the third month, the client's menstrual cycle had regulated to 29 days, marking a significant milestone in

	her hormonal health journey. Additionally, headaches became less severe and less frequent.
Additional Therapeutic Techniques:	The main recommendation for the client is to continue seed cycling in sync with her natural menstrual cycle. Additionally, tracking symptoms and changes in her well-being through a journal is vital for monitoring progress and making further adjustments if needed. The client encountered two headaches that didn't appear directly related to her menstrual cycle, and they were less severe compared to previous experiences. As a result, a decision was made to continue monitoring headaches for further insights and patterns.
Outcomes to Client's Health:	Over the course of 4 months, the client experienced notable improvements in her health, including the return of her menstrual cycle, healthier periods, and signs of ovulation. The client's skin health improved, and headaches became less severe and less frequent. The flexible approach, including adjusting the seed cycling protocol, allowed for tailoring to the client's needs, resulting in a holistic, well-rounded strategy for addressing her hormonal imbalances and overall well-being.

Nutritionist Case Study 2 – Anovulatory Cycles, Trying to Conceive

Client Background:	The client was TCC (Trying to Conceive) for 6 months. She struggled with irregular cycles, anovulatory cycles from time to time as well as a history of acne and eczema. Diet and lifestyle were poor, including high processed food, saturated fat and alcohol intake.
Integration:	Worked on improving her diet and lifestyle, moving toward the Mediterranean dietary pattern and removing alcohol whilst TTC. Together we worked on tracking her cycle, becoming more aware and in tune with her body and Basal Body Temperature (BBT) charting as well. During our 12 weeks together, the client was offered The Seed Cycle™ products and spoke to her about the benefits of seed cycling to help improve her menstrual cycle, hormones and fertility.
Progress and Changes:	The client used the seeds for the last 4 weeks of our time together. During the 12 weeks she saw an improvement in her skin, her eczema, menstrual cycle regulation and fell pregnant!
Client Feedback:	The client was excited to trial The Seed Cycle™ Phase 1 and 2 seeds and found it to be incredibly convenient and easy way to add more healthy fats and key fertility boosting nutrients into her diet.
Collaborative Approach:	Lifestyle - reduced/removed alcohol, improved sleep routine and quality, stress management, reduced exposure to toxins, increased gentle movement and reduced High Intensity

	Training (HIT).
	Diet - moved from highly processed, nutrient-poor diet to a wholefood, nutrient dense diet (med diet pattern) that included more veg, fruit, healthy fats, wholegrains, legumes, water. Also focused on dietary strategies to improve ovulation including adding in more seeds through The Seed Cycle™ products.
	Supplements were used to optimise nutrient levels in addition to food sources and help support her nervous system/stress response.
Conclusion:	The client was excited to trial The Seed Cycle™ Phase 1 and 2 seeds and found it to be an incredibly convenient and easy way to add more healthy fats and key fertility boosting nutrients into her diet. She would add these to yoghurt, overnight oats, smoothies, salads and soups. She found them so versatile as well.
	Throughout the time working together the client felt that her hormonal balance had improved, her skin had improved, and she fell pregnant naturally. The seeds made a great addition to the dietary approach, and she was so grateful for the opportunity to try them.

Practitioner Case Study 3 – PCOS

Client Background	32-year-old female with PCOS. Main symptoms were weight gain, hirsutism, heavy painful periods, headaches at ovulation, fatigue, bloating, significant cravings, difficulty sleeping (wakes multiple times nightly).
	She was on the pill to manage symptoms for years and worked with me to come off the pill in Feb 2023. After stopping she had irregular periods for about 3 months which are now back to 30ish day cycles.
	Blood tests showed high fasting insulin and glucose (insulin resistance), elevated liver enzymes, high triglycerides and cholesterol, high free testosterone which is the fraction of testosterone not bound to proteins. Post pill we have done some hormone testing showing low progesterone post ovulation (oestrogen normal levels but unopposed).
	Stressful lifestyle (mostly work), nil exercise. Struggles with consistency with diet and supplements. Lack of water intake (<1.5L). Previously tried 1200 calorie diet with Dietitian without success.
Integration:	After achieving consistency with blood sugar balancing meals and snacks and a move to predominantly wholefoods, we introduced seed cycling. The easiest and most enjoyable way she incorporated it was her daily snack of yoghurt, berries and seeds or a protein smoothie. I initially recommended The Seed Cycle™ to her, but she was buying her own seeds to begin with. Because of this she was

	inconsistent with it and would end up using whatever seeds she had (mostly flaxseed) for convenience rather than cycling them. Approx 4-5 months ago she ordered The Seed Cycle™ and has since been consistent with it approx. 95% of the time!
Progress and Changes:	Seed cycling has been really effective, especially since coming off the pill for her. Not only for the nutritional and therapeutic benefits but for her to reconnect to her menstrual cycle and body and understand her cyclical rhythms. It's helped her become more conscious of her nutrition overall and conscious of how she experiences each phase of her cycle. Over this time her menstrual cycles have gone from 45+ days in length to 30ish days. Headaches at ovulation have significantly reduced. Triglycerides and cholesterol have reduced significantly. Insulin has come down slightly but still more work to be done here with her diet. Sleep has improved dramatically. Weight loss has been slow, but weight gain has stopped as previously she was gaining weight monthly. No longer has painful or heavy periods. Cravings significantly reduced.
Client Feedback:	"I'm now consistent with my seed cycling because its super convenient" and "loves the scoop because I don't have to fuss around with making sure I've measured it out". "I feel confident knowing that the seeds are actually fresh (and not rancid oils), and I can easily access organic seeds that are otherwise hard to find."

Collaborative Approach:	Consistent macro balanced/blood sugar balanced meals and snacks (tried lower carb / carb cycling / Autoimmune Protocol (AIP) protocol for grain free to reduce insulin resistance but she struggled with it - we've got some mindset shifts around this to do) - Increased protein intake. - Started exercise, gym/weight 3-4x weekly plus walks. - Wholefoods and increased anti-inflammatory foods. - Seed cycling. - Meal prepping to avoid takeaway. - Prebiotics, probiotics and resistance starch + fibre diversity for gut. - move to low tox products. - Stress management practices - journalling, meditation, breathwork (not consistent yet) - Supplementation (has changed over time) but currently focused on insulin resistance/blood glucose management, liver support, reducing inflammation, sleep and nervous system support.
Conclusion:	This client has experienced significant improvements to her PCOS symptoms and blood markers overall, especially considering the impact of coming off the pill and supporting her body through the hormonal shifts that occur from that. She has made huge changes to her nutrition and lifestyle over time and continued with these changes where previously she would only stick to "diets" for short periods of time before going back to old habits. She has built a deeper awareness and

	connection to her body and her cycles and seed cycling has been the catalyst for this. This has helped her feel more confident in providing her body what it needs and knowing how to support her body to improve her health.

Nutritionist Case Study 4 – Irregular Periods, Mood, Pain and Hair Loss

Client Background	Age – 40 Lifestyle – Gluten free, eats a healthy diet. Exercises when she can - always looking for ways to improve her health. Health Concerns - Period = irregular, sometimes heavy, sometimes watery. Always accompanied with rage, bloating, pain, itching, hair loss & sugar cravings. Medical History - Carrier for Hemochromatosis, Gallbladder removal, follows Gluten free diet.
Integration:	Client had previously seen another practitioner who had diagnosed her with low progesterone and put her on Menstrocare (Supplement to boost progesterone naturally) As she was already on this, we introduced seed cycling to accompany this supplement but in the last cycle she decided to stop this and just do the seed cycling.
Progress and Changes:	Client is currently on 3rd month of seed cycling. Client has noticed period symptoms have settled - she has not needed to take any pain medication or use heat bags. Flow is heavy for 3 days and then spotting for final 2 days. Period has become regular. She has noticed less hair loss and noted that her hair is less greasy/smelly. Itching is still the same & sugar cravings still present. Biggest improvement has been her moods - she hasn't had any irrational anger/rage or uncontrolled sobbing. Sad moments are a few

	tears.
Client Feedback:	Really enjoying the product - has opted for the cookies & brownies mix to continue on for her 4th round.
Collaborative Approach:	Continued with Menstrocare for the first 2 cycles as she was already on this and then discussed stopping it and just using The Seed Cycle™ to see how she goes.
Conclusion:	Overall, the client has really enjoyed seed cycling - she has only missed a couple of days out of the 3 months. She is going to continue with it. She has found it has improved her cycle - making it more regular, less pain and her emotional well-being has improved significantly.

Chapter 8
Seed Cycling Benefits and How to Get Started

We have explored the origins, research, and science behind seed cycling, but you may still have many questions about the benefits, how to start, and how long it takes to work? You may be confused as to how to seed cycle if your menstrual cycle is irregular, or you are on the pill. This chapter will address your questions about seed cycling and help you feel confident to begin your practice. You will see how seed cycling seamlessly integrates the best of nutritional and naturopathic approaches, and I am excited for you to experience the benefits of seed cycling for yourself!

The Role of Seed Cycling in Wellness

Think of seed cycling as a form of menstrual biohacking—a holistic approach that harnesses the power of nature and science to optimise your hormonal health. By aligning specific nutrients with the natural fluctuations of your menstrual cycle, you can support your body's innate ability to regulate the key female sex hormones.

When we engage in the practice of seed cycling, we are connecting to the sisterhood of women who have used the power of nature to nurture and heal. The act of incorporating seeds into our daily lives is not just a wellness practice; it's a thread linking us to the feminine wisdom of the past.

Benefits of Seed Cycling

I have seen the incredible benefits firsthand with the thousands of customers who have seed cycled with us. Seed cycling offers a multitude of advantages that can dramatically enhance both your physical and emotional well-being. At its core, seed cycling aims to support hormonal balance by providing the body with specific nutrients needed for hormone production and metabolism. The benefits of seed cycling come from the nutrients in the seeds, as well as the cyclical rotation of the seeds, which help regulate estrogen and progesterone levels, having widespread effects on overall health and well-being.

Here's an expanded look at some of the researched and reported benefits:

> **Improved Skin Clarity**: The nutrients found in the seeds used in seed cycling, such as Omega-3 and Omega-6 fatty acids, Vitamin E, and zinc, can contribute to healthier skin. These nutrients may help reduce inflammation, regulate oil production, and support collagen production, leading to clearer and more radiant skin.
>
> **Clear Hormonal Acne**: Seed cycling can be a powerful tool in clearing hormonal acne by addressing its root cause. Hormonal acne often results from fluctuations in estrogen, progesterone, and androgens, which can trigger excess oil production and inflammation. Seed cycling helps regulate these hormone levels by providing essential nutrients and phytoestrogens that support the body's natural hormone balance. You can see our customers skin before and after seed cycling results on our website (www.theseedcycle.com.au) and social media (@the_seed_cycle).
>
> **Reduced PMS Symptoms**: Seed cycling is most well-known for its potential to reduce premenstrual syndrome (PMS) symptoms, bringing significant relief to many individuals. By promoting hormonal balance, seed cycling can help alleviate common PMS symptoms including bloating, breast tenderness, mood swings, and fatigue, leading to a more comfortable and enjoyable menstrual experience.

Regulating Menstrual Cycle: Seed cycling continues to be proven effective in regulating menstrual cycles, as evidenced by numerous testimonials from customers and practitioners. This practice helps align a woman's cycle closer to the average 28 days, a sign of balanced hormones and a healthy menstrual cycle. Irregular cycles often indicate underlying issues or hormonal imbalances, and it's crucial to understand and address these root causes, which can stem from various factors such as stress, diet, or underlying health conditions.

Enhanced Mood: Hormonal fluctuations, especially low progesterone production in the luteal phase, can significantly influence mood throughout the menstrual cycle, as well as during perimenopause and menopause. Seed cycling can help to stabilise mood by providing essential nutrients that aid in progesterone production. The Omega-3 fatty acids found in the seeds are particularly beneficial for brain health and may contribute to improved mood regulation. By encouraging the body to produce more progesterone, seed cycling can help mitigate mood swings and enhance overall emotional stability.

Weight Loss Support: Customers are often shocked to notice a reduction in weight when seed cycling. Let's break down how exactly seed cycling supports weight loss. The combination of healthy fats, fibre, and nutrients in the seeds can help regulate appetite, reduce sugar cravings, and promote feelings of fullness, which may support weight management efforts. Excess estrogen in the body can lead to belly fat accumulation, as this hormone promotes fat storage, particularly around the abdomen. Seed cycling aids in estrogen detoxification by providing lignans and phytoestrogens, which can help balance estrogen levels. Flaxseeds, for instance, contain lignans that support the liver's ability to process and eliminate excess estrogen. By promoting a healthier estrogen balance, seed cycling helps reduce the tendency for belly fat storage, thereby supporting overall weight management and a healthier body composition.

Increased Energy and Vitality: Balanced hormones contribute to increased energy levels and vitality throughout the menstrual cycle. By supporting healthy hormones, seed cycling can help reduce fatigue and enhance overall vitality, helping us feel more energised and productive. Additionally, seed cycling can help address nutrient deficiencies; the seeds are like nature's multivitamin, providing essential nutrients such as Omega-3 fatty acids, fibre, and various vitamins and minerals. Building up these depleted nutrients goes a long way in boosting energy levels and overall well-being.

Seed Cycling for Fertility: In Chinese herbology, seeds are traditionally used to support fertility, encapsulating the idea of using seeds to generate "seeds." Nutrition significantly impacts fertility, and the practice of seed cycling has been found to balance the two main female hormones affecting pregnancy, progesterone and estrogen. Seed cycling encourages healthy ovulation and regular cycles, and promotes healthy cervical mucus, all which support conception. By aligning nutritional intake with the body's hormonal needs, seed cycling helps create an optimal environment for fertility. Always consult with your health care professional, if you are struggling with infertility as there may be underlying issues that need to be addressed.

Reducing PCOS Symptoms: Seed cycling has been researched for its potential to reduce symptoms associated with Polycystic Ovary Syndrome (PCOS) and other hormonal imbalances. PCOS, characterised by irregular menstrual cycles, excess androgen levels, and ovarian cysts, can be particularly challenging to manage. The nutrients in seeds used in seed cycling, such as lignans and Omega-3 fatty acids, can support hormonal balance, reduce inflammation, and promote regular menstrual cycles. These benefits may help alleviate common PCOS symptoms, such as acne, hirsutism (the growth of excessive male-pattern hair in women after puberty), and weight gain. For more detailed information and research on how seed cycling can help manage PCOS symptoms, refer to Chapter 11.

It is important to note that the benefits of seed cycling can vary from person to person, and individual experiences may differ. Additionally, while many individuals may experience positive outcomes from seed cycling, it may not be effective for everyone. As with any dietary or lifestyle change, it is advisable to consult with a healthcare provider before starting seed cycling, especially if you have underlying health conditions or concerns. While mild hormonal imbalances may benefit greatly from eating seeds, seed cycling alone is not likely to solve more complex causes of infertility, like blocked tubes, or advanced endometriosis.

Understanding the Seed Cycling Phases

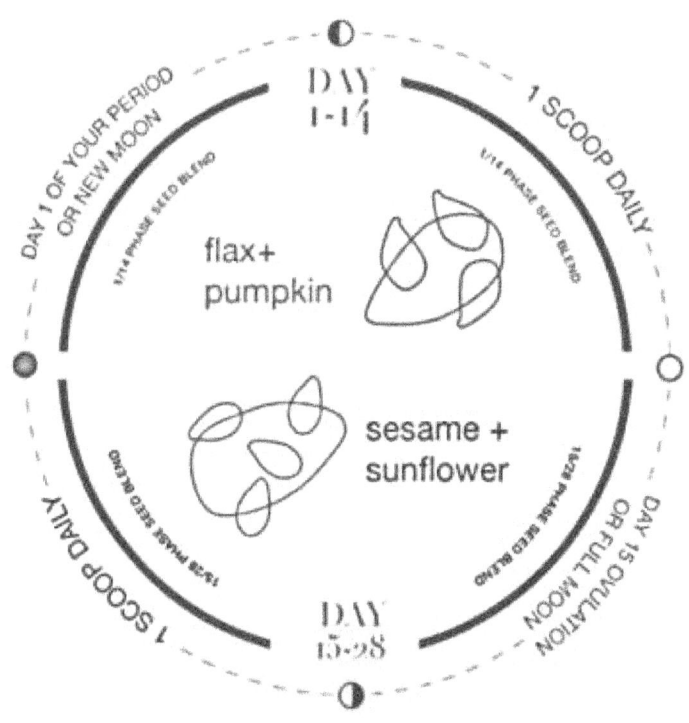

Figure 3 The Seed Cycle™ Diagram

Seed Cycling with the Menstrual Cycle Phases

Seed cycling aligns with the hormonal fluctuations and menstrual cycle phases we explored earlier - Menstrual, Follicular, Ovulation and Luteal.

A regular menstrual cycle typically lasts between 21 to 35 days, with the average cycle being around approximately 28 days. For the purposes of explaining seed cycling, we used the average 28-day cycle. While a cycle length outside the 21 to 35-day range may still be considered normal, irregularities in cycle length or consistency may warrant further investigation by a healthcare provider to rule out any underlying issues or hormonal imbalances.

Seed Cycling with The Moon Phases

The moon's phases can influence hormonal regulation within the body, including the release of neurohormones, sex hormones, and melatonin.

Seed cycling with the moon phases (lunar calendar) offers a gentle and natural way to encourage a cyclical rhythm when your own menstrual cycle is irregular or missing. As well as if you are transitioning off hormonal contraceptives, trying to conceive, pregnant or breastfeeding or navigating menopause.

By aligning with your body's innate wisdom and the rhythms of nature, specifically the moon phases, seed cycling can guide you back to a regular menstrual cycle or support key transitional periods of your life including puberty, pregnancy and menopause with grace and empowerment.

How to Seed Cycle

Now for the fun part—getting started with your seed cycling practice. Let's delve into how to start seed cycling with a step-by-step guide and tips for seamlessly incorporating it into your daily routine.

The phases of the menstrual cycle are divided into two phases for seed cycling:

The Seed Cycle™ Phase 1 - Menstrual and Follicular (Days 1–14)

> **Seeds to Consume:** Organic Ground Pumpkin Seeds and Organic Ground Flaxseeds.

> **Key Focus:** Support rising estrogen levels, essential for regulating the menstrual cycle.

The Seed Cycle™ Phase 2: Ovulation and Luteal (Days 15–28)

> **Seeds to Consume:** Organic ground, Sesame Seeds and Organic Ground Sunflower Seeds.
>
> **Key Focus:** Support hormone balance and overall well-being during the luteal phase.

Seed Cycling with Irregular or Missing Cycles and Menopause:

> The Seed Cycle™ Phase 1: Begins on the first day of the **new moon**, consuming pumpkin seeds and flaxseeds.
>
> The Seed Cycle™ Phase 2: Transitions to the **full moon**, consuming sesame seeds and sunflower seeds.
>
> **Key Focus:** Tapping into the natural rhythms of the lunar cycle can guide seed consumption and hormonal balancing, providing a natural way to encourage a cyclical rhythm.

How to Seed Cycle Summary – Menstrual Cycle or aligning with the Moon Phases

Phase	Days (Approx.)	Seeds	Benefits
Menstrual and Follicular	1–14	Pumpkin Seeds, Flaxseeds	Omega-3 fatty acids promote hormone production, lignans modulate estrogen levels, support heathy iron levels.
Ovulation and Luteal	15–28	Sesame Seeds, Sunflower Seeds	Omega-6 fatty acids support hormone synthesis, lignans help regulate estrogen levels, and Vitamin E provides antioxidant protection.
Irregular/Missing Cycles & Menopause (Lunar calendar)	New Moon (Days 1–14)	Pumpkin Seeds, Flaxseeds	Aligns with lunar rhythms, supporting hormonal balance through Omega-3s, lignans, and iron.
	Full Moon (Days 15–28)	Sesame Seeds, Sunflower Seeds	Omega-6 fatty acids, lignans, and Vitamin E continue to support hormone balance.

Therapeutic Dosage for Seed Cycling

Adhering to the therapeutic dosage for seed cycling is a crucial part of the practice. Here is a detailed look at the recommended dosage and usage:

Traditional and Recommended Usage:

> **Dosage:** 1 tablespoon of each seed daily, ground.
>
> **Method:** Correspond with the phases of your menstrual cycle or lunar calendar

Menstrual Cycle or Lunar Calendar	Seeds	Dosage (Daily)
Follicular Phase (Day 1-14) or New Moon	Organic Flaxseeds, Organic Pumpkin Seeds	1 tablespoon each day, ground
Luteal Phase (Day 15-28) or Full Moon	Organic Sesame seeds, Organic Sunflower Seeds	1 tablespoon each day, ground

Additional Information:

Historical Context: Traditional Ayurvedic and Chinese medicine advocate for 1 tablespoon of each seed, depending on the current phase of the menstrual cycle. This practice aligns with natural rhythms to support hormonal balance.

Research and Expert Endorsement: While the original research behind seed cycling is challenging to pinpoint, current hormone experts such as Dr. Jolene Brighton follow this dosage protocol, affirming its efficacy.

Consumption Tips: Seeds can be consumed at any time of day, ideally with food. They can be added to:

- Yoghurt
- Salads

- Soups
- Smoothies
- Recipes such as bliss balls (See Chapter 12 for Seed Cycling Recipes)

Using The Seed Cycle™ Products

When I launched The Seed Cycle™, my goal was to simplify seed cycling for my clients by offering products that are both convenient and of the highest quality. This mission remains at the core of what we do. We are dedicated to using only certified organic ingredients and ensuring their freshness and nutrient integrity. To uphold these standards, we conduct rigorous third-party testing on our products to check for potency, mould, heavy metals, and other contaminants. This unwavering commitment to quality means that my customers always receive the most effective and safe seed cycling products available.

Our seeds come ground which we do in small batches to ensure stability and nutrient quality of the seeds.

Tips for incorporating seed cycling into daily routines

Incorporating seed cycling into your daily routine can be a simple and enjoyable process with a few helpful tips. One way to seamlessly integrate seed cycling is by incorporating seeds into your meals and snacks. You can sprinkle Seed Cycle Phase 1 or 2 onto your morning porridge, yoghurt or add them to smoothies for an extra nutrient boost. For a savoury option for the seeds can be added into salads, soups, or stir-fries, they add such a great texture and flavour.

The Seed Cycle™ Bake Mixes and Seed Cycling + Protein are convenient alternatives to traditional seed cycling blends, providing the correct dosage of cycling seeds in an easy, delicious form. When using these products as directed, there's no need to add extra ground seeds to your diet. The bake mixes, which are simple to prepare with just eggs and oil (I love using avocado oil for brownies and coconut oil for biscuits), also come in vegan options.

These bake mixes have a meaningful backstory. When my sister-in-law came off the pill, she faced hormonal acne and her period hadn't returned. Finding it hard to incorporate the seeds into her routine, I suggested hiding them in a snack, like a brownie. Inspired, I created healthy, dairy-free, gluten-free, and refined sugar-free brownies and biscuits. She loved them, and the best part? Her skin improved, and her period came back. It was my first firsthand seed cycling success story.

Recently, we introduced Seed Cycling + Protein mixes—an innovative, world-first seed cycling protein blend, offering complete nutritional and hormonal support over a one-month cycle. These blends feature Organic Inca Inchi and Hemp Protein for a full amino acid profile, along with Camu Camu for a rich dose of Vitamin C, enhancing immune support. Customers love the convenience of integrating seed cycling seamlessly into their routine, along with the extra boost of protein and vital nutrients these products provide.

Consistency Equals Results

While some benefits may be noticed within the first month of seed cycling, more substantial changes, such as regular menstrual cycles and relief from menopause symptoms, typically require consistent practice over 3 to 4 months. It's essential to continue seed cycling beyond this period to maintain optimal hormone balance.

When getting started with your seed cycling routine it might help to set a reminder or alarm on your phone to help you stay consistent with seed cycling, ensuring that you don't miss a day. By incorporating these simple strategies into your daily routine, you can effectively support your hormonal health with seed cycling while enjoying delicious and nutritious meals and snacks.

Postpartum Hormones and Seed Cycling

After childbirth, progesterone drops off almost immediately after delivering the placenta, while prolactin remains elevated to support breastfeeding. Your ovaries will not start creating progesterone again until your first menstrual cycle, potentially creating a temporary hormonal imbalance. Seed cycling post-partum can help soften the emotional changes that can occur due to this hormonal shift.

At around two to three months postpartum, your hormones begin to reset to pre-pregnancy levels, but you may still experience hormonal changes even months after your baby's birth. If you've experienced a hormone imbalance before pregnancy, there's a higher likelihood you'll experience it again once your pregnancy hormones subside.

Signs of Postpartum Hormonal Imbalance

Sometimes, pregnancy and childbirth can cause your hormones to become a bit out of balance. Symptoms of postpartum hormonal imbalance can include:

- Chronic fatigue
- Anxiety and depression
- Weight gain
- Cysts or fibroids
- Low libido

Customers who have seed cycled postpartum have reported benefits such as:

- Little to no postpartum acne and healthier-looking skin
- Better sleep (apart from waking up for the baby)
- More stable mood

Seed Cycling Postpartum When Menstrual Cycle Has Not Returned

If your menstrual cycle has not yet returned or is irregular postpartum, it's recommended to use the phases of the moon as a guide to cycle dates. This method allows for the harmonisation of hormonal balance and the benefits of seed cycling.

Contraindications for Seed Cycling

There are a few contraindications to consider when practicing seed cycling. If an individual has a seed allergy—such as an allergy to sesame seeds—they should avoid that specific seed. In cases where only one seed causes an allergic reaction, it's possible to double up on the other seed used in that phase. For example, if you're allergic to sesame seeds, you could increase the dosage of sunflower seeds during the luteal phase

For individuals with irritable bowel syndrome (IBS) or digestive sensitivities, the fibre and lignan content in seeds can cause bloating or stomach upset. This can also be the case for those who are consuming an ultra-processed diet with little fibre. It's recommended to start with half a dose and gradually increase it to allow the digestive system to adapt.

Additionally, those with histamine intolerance may experience reactions to certain seeds, particularly flax and sesame, which can act as histamine triggers. Histamine intolerance occurs when the body has difficulty breaking down histamine, resulting in symptoms such as headaches, hives, or digestive issues. For individuals with histamine issues, starting with half a dose and working with a healthcare practitioner is essential to ensure proper tolerance and adjustment.

Reducing Antinutrients in Seed Cycling

The seed cycling seeds contain small amounts of antinutrients like phytic acid which can hinder the absorption of important minerals such as calcium, magnesium, and zinc. Although these antinutrients are naturally present in many plant-based foods, they serve a protective function for the plant but may reduce nutrient availability in our diets. While lectins, another type of antinutrient, are commonly found in beans and grains, the seeds used in seed cycling contain very low levels of lectins, making them less of a concern. Nonetheless, for those with sensitive digestion, addressing the presence of these antinutrients is important to ensure the body can fully absorb the beneficial nutrients in the seeds.

At The Seed Cycle™, we use a cold-milling process to grind the seeds, which not only preserves the delicate nutrients but also helps reduce the effects of antinutrients like phytic acid and lectins. Cold milling ensures that the seeds are broken down in a way that maintains their nutrient integrity while making them easier to digest and absorb. Grinding the seeds also increases their surface area, which makes it easier for the body to break down the seeds and access the healthy fats, fibre, and phytoestrogens they provide. This process helps reduce potential digestive discomfort and enhances the nutritional benefits of seed cycling, ensuring you get the most out of each phase.

Oil Cycling for Added Support to Seed Cycling

In recent years, oil cycling has gained attention as a valuable addition to the seed cycling practice, particularly within online naturopathic and health communities. Many practitioners and enthusiasts have begun to explore how this approach can support seed cycling and enhance hormonal balance.

Oil cycling is a complementary practice to seed cycling, further enhancing hormonal balance by introducing targeted fats rich in essential fatty acids. During the follicular phase (from menstruation to ovulation), the body benefits from Omega-3 fatty acids, particularly DHA (Docosahexaenoic acid) and EPA (Eicosapentaenoic acid), which can be sourced from marine algae oil. These essential fatty acids support estrogen production, reduce inflammation, and contribute to overall hormonal health. Marine algae oil, a plant-based alternative to fish oil, offers the same benefits without environmental contaminants that can be found in fish oils, making it ideal for vegans and those seeking clean, sustainable options.

For the luteal phase (from ovulation to menstruation), evening primrose oil is highly beneficial due to its high content of gamma-linolenic acid (GLA). GLA helps balance progesterone levels, alleviates PMS symptoms, and supports overall reproductive health. The practice of oil cycling, much like seed cycling, is rooted in Functional Nutrition, focusing on nourishing the body in alignment with hormonal shifts. While oil cycling alongside seed cycling is a relatively new concept in natural health, it draws from ancient principles of using food as medicine to support the body's natural rhythms.

Let's go through some of the seed cycling frequently asked questions:

When do I start seed cycling?

Starting seed cycling is a flexible process that can be initiated at any point in your menstrual cycle. You don't have to wait until the first day of your period or a new moon to begin seed cycling.

> For example:
>
> Imagine you are on day 5 of your menstrual cycle. In this scenario, you can kickstart your seed cycling journey by starting with Phase 1 - flaxseeds and pumpkin seeds. You would continue consuming Phase 1 for the next 9 days until you reach day 14 of your cycle or ovulation.

Once you reach day 15 or ovulation, it's time to transition to Phase 2 – sunflower and sesame seeds. After completing Phase 2, you would switch back to Phase 1 on the first day of your next cycle, which corresponds to day 1 of your period.

How do I know if I have ovulated?

Ovulation, the process in which a mature egg is released from the ovary, typically occurs around the midpoint of the menstrual cycle in women with regular cycles. There are several signs and symptoms that can help you identify when you're ovulating.

One of the most common indicators of ovulation is changes in cervical mucus. As ovulation approaches, cervical mucus typically becomes clear, slippery, and stretchy, resembling the consistency of egg whites. This fertile-quality cervical mucus facilitates sperm survival and transportation, making it easier for conception to occur.

Another sign of ovulation is an increase in basal body temperature (BBT). Tracking your BBT with a basal body thermometer can help you identify the slight rise in temperature that occurs after ovulation due to increased progesterone levels. This temperature shift usually occurs one to two days after ovulation and can help confirm that ovulation has occurred.

For the purposes of seed cycling, we recommend tracking your cycle and paying attention to cervical mucus changes to signal when to switch to Phase 2. If you are not 100% sure if you've ovulated – switch anyway to Phase 2. Estimating is enough, and we don't want it to be something you feel stressed about.

If you have irregular cycles or difficulty pinpointing ovulation, consider consulting with a healthcare provider for personalised guidance and support. Over time, you will learn the signals, and the switch will become intuitive and easy.

Why do the seeds have to be ground?

When seed cycling, it's important to consume ground seeds as opposed to whole seeds for a few reasons:

First, consuming ground seeds makes it easier for the body to absorb the nutrients contained in the seeds. Whole seeds have a hard outer shell that can be difficult for the body to break down, which can limit the amount of nutrients that are absorbed. Ground seeds, on the other hand, have a larger surface area, making it easier for the body to access the nutrients contained within them.

Second, ground seeds are easier to digest than whole seeds because they break down more efficiently in the digestive system, allowing better absorption of nutrients. This process can also help reduce the impact of antinutrients—compounds found in certain plants that can interfere with the absorption of essential minerals like calcium, magnesium, and zinc.

Can I seed cycle if I am on the Pill or Hormone Replacement Therapy (HRT)?

Seed cycling can be incorporated into your routine even if you are taking the oral contraceptive pill or hormone replacement therapy (HRT). It will not negatively affect your medication, and you can still benefit from the nutrient-rich properties of seeds. Seeds contain tryptophan, an essential amino acid that the body uses to produce serotonin (the happy hormone) and melatonin (the sleep hormone). This can help improve sleep quality and stabilise mood. The additional support from seed cycling can help in achieving a more balanced hormonal state, potentially alleviating symptoms like bloating and fatigue.

You can also align your seed cycling practice with the moon phases—using Phase 1 during the new moon and Phase 2 during the full moon—to further connect with natural rhythms. Incorporating seed cycling alongside your medication regimen can enhance your health and well-being, offering a natural complement to your existing treatments.

Can I seed cycle if have had a hysterectomy?

Yes, you can still benefit from seed cycling even if you have had a hysterectomy. While a hysterectomy involves the removal of the uterus, it does not necessarily affect your hormone production if your ovaries remain intact. Seed cycling can help support overall hormonal balance, which is beneficial for many aspects of health, even after a hysterectomy.

Seed cycling helps the body mimic a regular menstrual cycle by providing the necessary nutrients to support the phases of hormone production. This is especially important for maintaining hormonal equilibrium and reducing symptoms associated with hormone imbalances. Additionally, seed cycling can assist the body in eliminating xenoestrogens from the environment, which are synthetic compounds that mimic estrogen and can disrupt normal hormone function.

To practice seed cycling without a menstrual cycle, you can follow the moon phases.

How long before I see results?

Many of our customers report experiencing noticeable benefits within the initial month of seed cycling, such as improved skin clarity and enhanced digestion.

For more substantial and significant changes, including regular menstrual cycles, relief from PMS symptoms, and alleviation of menopause symptoms, it typically takes around three to four months of consistent seed cycling.

It's helpful to continue seed cycling beyond this to maintain optimal hormone balance. Please note all results are very individual.

How long do I continue seed cycling?

It can be part of your daily routine long term to support your body as you move through all the stages of life. There is no need to stop or take a break as it is all natural.

Can I seed cycle while pregnant and breastfeeding?

Incorporating seed cycling with the moon phases during pregnancy can provide a great source of nutrients. The nutrient-dense seeds offer essential vitamins, minerals, and healthy fats necessary for a healthy pregnancy and can also be extremely beneficial post-partum.

Can men seed cycle?

Yes! Men can benefit from the nutrients in these seeds to support overall health. The nutrients in the seeds can be particularly supportive for men's prostate health. Pumpkin seeds are rich in zinc, supporting healthy sperm, prostate health, and testosterone levels. Flaxseeds contain lignans that balance estrogen levels and have anti-inflammatory properties. Sesame seeds provide lignans and healthy fats, improving serum lipids, blood pressure, and inflammatory markers. Sunflower seeds are high in vitamin E, protecting cells from oxidative damage and reducing inflammation.

Men can follow the moon phases for seed cycling or have all four seeds each day. While men do have lower estrogen levels than women, balanced estrogen is important for reproductive, bone, and cognitive health. To be honest, I am yet to meet a man who is seed cycling with the phases of the moon, I can tell you my husband regularly enjoys the Seed Cycling + Protein and The Seed Cycle™ Biscuits and Brownies

Chapter 9
Seed Cycling for PMS, the Pill and Teens

In this chapter, we delve into the complexities of Premenstrual Syndrome (PMS), shedding light on the misconception that PMS is normal. While common, PMS should not be considered a natural part of the menstrual cycle. Instead, it often signifies underlying hormonal imbalances that warrant attention and support.

We will explore why seed cycling is emerging as a natural and gentle approach to alleviate premenstrual symptoms, offering insights into its benefits in promoting hormonal harmony.

Additionally, we discuss how seed cycling can serve as a valuable tool in preparing the body for transitioning off birth control as well as empowering teens to take charge of their hormonal health and well-being.

Through understanding the principles and practices of seed cycling, adolescents can cultivate a deeper connection with their bodies and support their journey towards hormonal balance and vitality.

Understanding PMS

PMS or period problems are common experiences for many women, yet they are often misunderstood and mismanaged. Most women I speak to say they get some premenstrual symptoms, such as bloating, headaches, and moodiness. Understanding the nature of PMS and its causes can help us take control of our menstrual health and reduce symptoms effectively.

The Nature of PMS

PMS encompasses a variety of physical and emotional symptoms that occur after ovulation and before menstruation. Symptoms can range from mild to severe, and for some, they can be debilitating. The fluctuation of hormones, particularly estrogen and progesterone, is a natural part of the menstrual cycle. However, when these fluctuations are extreme, they can lead to PMS or even Premenstrual Dysphoric Disorder (PMDD), a severe form of PMS.

Symptoms of PMS

PMS symptoms vary widely but typically include physical and emotional symptoms, which can significantly impact daily activities and quality of life.

Physical Symptoms:

- Swollen or tender breasts
- Bloating or gassiness
- Cramping
- Headaches or backaches
- Constipation or diarrhea
- Clumsiness
- Sensitivity to noise or light

Emotional Symptoms:

- Irritability or hostility
- Fatigue
- Sleep disturbances
- Appetite changes or food cravings
- Difficulty concentrating
- Anxiety or tension
- Depression or sadness
- Mood swings

Misconceptions and Mismanagement

As women, we may have been told that periods are a curse and that the pain, headaches, and PMS are simply things we must endure, 'it's part of being a woman'. This narrative is pervasive and harmful, leading many women to believe that suffering through these symptoms is a normal part of life. However, these symptoms are signs of hormonal imbalances and should not be ignored or accepted as the norm.

Many women report frustrating experiences when seeking help from their doctors for PMS. They are frequently prescribed the pill or dismissed, this response not only fails to address the underlying issues but also perpetuates the cycle of pain and discomfort.

Causes of PMS

Several factors contribute to PMS, which is a complex condition influenced by hormonal fluctuations, lifestyle habits, and individual physiological responses. Understanding these underlying causes can help in managing the symptoms effectively and improving overall well-being.

The main contributing factors include:

Hormonal Imbalances

> **Estrogen Excess**: Elevated estrogen levels relative to progesterone, known as estrogen dominance, can lead to common PMS symptoms such as irritability, mood swings, and breast tenderness. This imbalance is often due to various factors, including poor liver detoxification, stress, or insulin resistance.
>
> **Progesterone Fluctuations**: Progesterone, a calming hormone, interacts with GABA (gamma-aminobutyric acid) receptors—proteins in the brain that respond to GABA, the main inhibitory neurotransmitter—helping to calm the nervous system and regulate anxiety, relaxation, and sleep.
>
> Low or fluctuating progesterone levels can increase sensitivity to stress, leading to symptoms like irritability, anxiety, and sleep disturbances.

Inflammatory Markers

Chronic inflammation can disrupt the body's natural hormonal balance, impacting ovulation and overall hormone health.

Impact on Ovulation: Inflammatory markers, such as C-reactive protein (CRP), can interfere with regular ovulation by disrupting the hormonal signals that trigger egg release. This can lead to irregular ovulation and lower progesterone levels, affecting the menstrual cycle.

Hormone Detoxification: Inflammation also hampers the body's ability to process and eliminate hormones, especially estrogen. When liver function or gut health is compromised, estrogen can build up, leading to symptoms of estrogen dominance like intense PMS, bloating, and mood swings.

In essence, chronic inflammation can throw off hormonal rhythms, making cycles irregular and PMS symptoms worse.

Other Factors Contributing to PMS

Nutritional Deficiencies: Low levels of magnesium, calcium, vitamin D, and B vitamins are commonly linked with more severe PMS symptoms like fatigue, headaches, and mood swings.

Stress and Cortisol Dysregulation: Chronic stress raises cortisol levels, which can disturb hormonal balance by decreasing progesterone and exacerbating estrogen dominance, intensifying PMS symptoms.

Gut Health and Microbiome: The gut microbiota plays a key role in estrogen metabolism. Dysbiosis, or imbalance in gut bacteria, can lead to improper estrogen recirculation, contributing to hormonal imbalance and PMS.

Endocrine-Disrupting Chemicals (EDCs): EDCs, commonly found in plastics, personal care products, and household items, can mimic or interfere with natural hormones, disrupting the delicate balance of estrogen and progesterone, leading to worsened PMS symptoms.

Addressing these factors holistically can help in alleviating PMS symptoms and restoring hormonal balance.

Seed Cycling for PMS

Effective management of PMS involves addressing its root causes rather than just masking symptoms. The practise of seed cycling has gained attention for its effectiveness in reducing PMS symptoms.

> **Impact on Ovulation**: Inflammatory markers, such as C-reactive protein (CRP), can interfere with regular
>
> ovulation by disrupting the hormonal signals that trigger egg release. This can lead to irregular ovulation and lower progesterone levels, affecting the menstrual cycle.
>
> **Hormone Detoxification**: Inflammation also hampers the body's ability to process and eliminate hormones, especially estrogen. When liver function or gut health is compromised, estrogen can build up, leading to symptoms of estrogen dominance like intense PMS, bloating, and mood swings.

I have had many women share their positive seed cycling experiences with me regarding the efficacy the seeds have had on their bodies to reduce PMS:

> *"I've been using Seed Cycle for about 4 months. Honestly, I have been so impressed with how effective they have been. My cycles have gone from 35 days to 28, but the main thing I have been so impressed with is that my periods are now so calming*
>
> *- I have practically no pain whatsoever. I literally feel a sense of peace, letting go & calm when I have my period - which is beautiful and definitely not what I have felt in the past. Plus, they are super convenient to add into so many different meals."*
> – Megan G.

Others have shared that they have experienced reductions in symptoms such as irritability, headaches, and food cravings.

Working with a practitioner can help you uncover the root causes of your PMS and develop a personalised strategy that aligns with your unique needs. Incorporating seed cycling into this comprehensive plan can be a powerful tool for restoring balance.

While it may take up to three months to see significant improvements, the journey towards understanding your body better and enhancing your health is well worth the effort.

Additional Strategies for PMS Relief

> **Limit Ultra-Processed Foods and Alcohol:** These can disrupt hormonal balance. Instead, focus on whole, nutrient-dense foods.
>
> **Ensure Adequate Iodine Intake**: Iodine stabilises estrogen receptors and supports thyroid function. Include iodine-rich foods like seaweed and fish.
>
> **Improve Gut Health:** A balanced gut microbiome aids estrogen metabolism. Incorporate probiotics and fibre-rich foods to support gut health.
>
> **Minimise Endocrine Disrupting Chemicals (EDCs):** Found in many products, EDCs can upset hormone balance. Choose natural products, use glass or stainless steel instead of plastic, and favour fresh foods over processed options.
>
> **Nervous System:** Manage stress through practices like yoga, meditation, or mindfulness.

Body Literacy

Value your hormones, recognising that both estrogen and progesterone play crucial roles in overall health. Support natural hormone fluctuations rather than suppress them with hormonal birth control.

Track your menstrual cycle to understand the different phases and how they affect your symptoms. Recognising the phase you're in can help tailor your approach to managing PMS and support overall hormonal health.

In understanding and honouring our cycles, we reclaim an aspect of sisterhood that is uniquely feminine.

Transitioning off the Pill: How Seed Cycling Can Help

When coming off the pill and other hormonal contraceptives, many women experience a range of symptoms as their bodies readjust to natural hormone production. This period can be marked by a resurgence of hormonal acne, irregular menstrual cycles, mood swings, and even significant menstrual pain and discomfort.

The synthetic hormones in birth control pills can mask underlying issues, and once these hormones are no longer present, any imbalances or health concerns may become more pronounced. In addressing these concerns, seed cycling emerges as a potentially beneficial strategy.

Post-Birth Control Syndrome (PBCS)

Post-Birth Control Syndrome (PBCS) is a collection of symptoms that some women experience after discontinuing hormonal birth control. This syndrome encompasses a wide range of physical and emotional challenges, including irregular menstrual cycles, severe hormonal acne, mood swings, anxiety, depression, and significant changes in libido.

The synthetic hormones found in birth control pills suppress the body's natural hormonal production, and when these external hormones are withdrawn, the body can struggle to establish its own hormonal balance. This period of readjustment can reveal underlying hormonal imbalances that were previously masked by the pill. Addressing PBCS requires a holistic approach and often requires the help of health care professionals.

Dr. Jolene Brighten, a leading expert in post-birth control syndrome shares that seed cycling is an effective way to support hormone balance, particularly for women who are coming off the pill. She has written extensively about the benefits of seed cycling and how it can be used to help regulate the menstrual cycle and support fertility.

It would be valuable to see more formal studies conducted specifically on the effectiveness of seed cycling for PBCS. As a company, we are working to gather documented case studies to better understand its potential impact. Anecdotally, we've heard from numerous customers who have noticed significant improvements in their PBCS symptoms after incorporating seed cycling into their routine. Given the way seed cycling works—by providing essential nutrients like zinc, magnesium, and lignans, which help regulate estrogen and progesterone levels—it is exciting to think that it could be more widely used to support women transitioning off hormonal birth control. Seed cycling may offer a natural solution to help restore the body's hormonal balance and alleviate the distressing symptoms associated with PBCS, such as irregular cycles, mood swings, and acne.

Benefits of Seed Cycling While on Hormonal Birth Control

In addition to seed cycling being beneficial for transitioning off hormonal birth control, it can also provide support while still using it, including:

> **Gut Health:** Seeds are rich in prebiotic fibre, which supports a healthy gut. Research indicates that oral contraceptives can negatively affect gut flora and disrupt estrogen metabolism. By incorporating seeds into your routine, you help maintain a balanced gut microbiome.
>
> **Nutrient Support:** Birth control pills can deplete essential nutrients such as riboflavin, B6, B12, folic acid, Vitamin C, magnesium, and zinc. Seed cycling provides a natural way to replenish these vital nutrients through your diet. *Please note: These nutrient depletions can lead to various health issues, making it important to monitor your nutrient intake and consult with a practitioner for proper guidance.*
>
> **Building a Relationship with Your Cycle:** Even though you're not ovulating or experiencing a natural menstrual cycle while on birth control, seed cycling offers a valuable opportunity to establish a connection with your cycle. This practice can be incredibly beneficial when you decide to transition off birth control, making the adjustment smoother and more intuitive.

Seed Cycling Protocol for Transitioning Off the Pill

Starting seed cycling 2-3 months before getting off the pill can be beneficial as it can help to prepare the body for the changes that will occur as hormone levels start to fluctuate naturally again. By supporting hormonal balance through seed cycling, women may be able to mitigate some of the potential side effects of coming off the pill, such as acne, mood changes, and irregular periods.

While on the pill it is recommended to seed cycle with the Lunar calendar or moon phases as this mimics a healthy menstrual cycle. (See Chapter 8 instructions for seed cycling with the moon phases)

Continue seed cycling after discontinuing the pill with the moon phases and once your menstrual cycle returns and is regular you can switch to seed cycling with your own cycle. This will help to support the body's ongoing hormonal balance.

Other important things to do when preparing your body naturally to get off the pill include:

Talk to your health care practitioner and ask them to help guide you with the transition.

Focus on a healthy diet. A healthy diet is essential for supporting your body as you transition off the pill. Focus on eating whole foods that are rich in nutrients, such as fruits, vegetables, whole grains, and lean proteins. Avoid processed foods, refined sugars, and unhealthy fats, which can disrupt your hormones and lead to inflammation.

Get enough sleep. Sleep is critical for hormonal balance. Aim for seven to eight hours of sleep each night to support your body as it adjusts to the changes.

Manage stress. Stress can impact your hormones and make it more difficult for your body to adjust to the changes associated with coming off the pill. Find healthy ways to manage stress, such as through exercise, meditation, or journaling.

Seed Cycling with the Mini-Pill, IUDs, and More

So far, we have primarily focused on the pill and its side effects, as well as how seed cycling can help mitigate these. However, seed cycling can also play a significant role in supporting those using other forms of birth control, such as the mini-pill, Mirena IUD (Intrauterine Device), copper IUD, and other hormonal IUDs.

The Mini-Pill contains only progestin (synthetic form of progesterone), which can alter cervical mucus and thin the uterine lining to prevent pregnancy. The Mirena IUD releases a small amount of progestin directly into the uterus, thickening the cervical mucus and thinning the lining, while also sometimes suppressing ovulation. The copper IUD, on the other hand, is a non-hormonal method that releases copper ions to create an inhospitable environment for sperm, preventing fertilisation.

These methods can lead to side effects such as irregular bleeding, mood swings, and changes in skin health.

They may also deplete essential nutrients, though the specific impact can vary. Factors such as individual physiology, duration of use, and dosage influence this depletion. Consulting with a healthcare provider to monitor nutrient levels and address potential deficiencies is crucial. Seed cycling offers a dual benefit, providing essential nutrients and aligning with the natural hormonal fluctuations of the menstrual cycle, making seed cycling a beneficial addition to any birth control regimen.

In conclusion, coming off the pill can be a complex process, but by using seed cycling and adopting healthy lifestyle habits, you can support your body's natural hormone balance. Remember to talk to a health care provider before making any changes to your birth control regimen and be patient with yourself as your body adjusts to the changes.

Teens and Puberty

Menstrual cycles typically begin during puberty, around the ages of 10 to 15 years old, marking a significant transition for girls. During this time, it can take several years for these cycles to mature and become regular. In this maturation process, many girls might experience a range of symptoms similar to those of PCOS, such as irregular periods, acne, and excess hair growth, as well as other PMS related issues like cramps, mood swings, hormonal acne and bloating.

This time can be particularly challenging and confusing for many teens. The natural hormonal fluctuations are often compounded by external factors such as stress from school and social pressures. The modern diet containing ultra processed foods, can also negatively impact hormonal balance, exacerbating symptoms. Additionally, environmental toxins found in everyday products can disrupt the endocrine system, further adding to the hormonal imbalances.

An alarming trend has seen the significant increase in young girls purchasing trending skincare and makeup products that contain active ingredients often full of endocrine-disrupting chemicals (EDCs). While these products promise clear skin and beauty, they can unknowingly contribute to hormonal symptoms. The presence of EDCs in these products can interfere with the body's natural hormone regulation, making conditions like acne, irregular cycles, and other PMS symptoms worse.

Addressing these issues involves educating young girls about the natural maturation of their menstrual cycles and the impact of diet, lifestyle, and environmental factors on their hormonal health. Encouraging healthier eating habits, reducing exposure to harmful chemicals, and managing stress can help mitigate these symptoms. Additionally, promoting the use of natural and safe skincare and beauty products can play a crucial role in supporting hormonal balance during these formative years.

Teens and the Pill

Teenage girls are often taken to doctors for the symptoms discussed above. Unfortunately, the common response from healthcare providers is to prescribe hormonal birth control. However, this approach does not address the root cause of the hormonal imbalances and often merely acts as a band aid solution.

By suppressing the menstrual cycle with synthetic hormones like the pill, it prevents the natural maturation process of the cycle. Once off the medication, individuals may find themselves facing even worse symptoms than before, as their bodies have not had the opportunity to mature and regulate hormones naturally. This phenomenon is why many women struggle immensely when coming off the pill, experiencing hormonal acne breakouts like those in their teenage years, even though they may be in their 30s or older.

I acknowledge that some teens and beyond are going on the pill for contraception, which is very different from being put on the pill as a solution for hormonal issues. Researching contraception methods that will work for you is important for making an informed decision. Many women are turning to using FAM (Fertility Awareness Method).

FAM offers a non-hormonal contraception alternative with comparable effectiveness when used correctly. Studies have shown that with proper education and diligent tracking, FAM can be up to 99.6% effective in preventing pregnancy, like the effectiveness of the pill. However, it's crucial to emphasise that consistency and accuracy in tracking menstrual cycles are paramount for FAM's success. While the pill offers immediate suppression of ovulation, FAM relies on understanding fertility patterns and abstaining or using barrier methods during fertile days.

I highly recommend working with a FAM practitioner (The Seed Cycle™ Directory in the resources section of the book has a list of recommended practitioners). By providing education and support, working with a practitioner can help you or a loved one make informed choices about your or their contraceptive options.

Seed Cycling for Teens

Seed cycling can be a beneficial and natural way for teens to help regulate their menstrual cycles and manage hormonal symptoms. For teens experiencing irregular periods, acne, and other PMS symptoms, seed cycling offers a holistic approach to manage these issues.

Introducing seed cycling to teens can help regulate their cycles but also provides a beautiful introduction to the concept of food as medicine. Understanding how different foods can impact their health empowers teens to make healthier choices and become more attuned to their bodies. By following a seed cycling regimen, teens can gain insights into their menstrual phases, learning to recognise and appreciate the natural rhythms of their bodies.

Moreover, seed cycling can help teens avoid the need for hormonal contraceptives, like the pill, for symptom management. By supporting the body's natural hormone production and balance, seed cycling addresses the root cause of hormonal imbalances rather than just masking the symptoms. This approach can lead to long-term health benefits and a deeper understanding of one's menstrual health.

Teens can start seed cycling to support hormonal balance and menstrual health. If a teen's menstrual cycle is regular, they can follow the phases of their cycle: Phase 1 begins on day 1 of bleeding (menstrual phase) and continues until around day 15 or ovulation (follicular phase), while

Phase 2 begins around day 15 (ovulation) and continues until the start of their next period (luteal phase).

However, for most teens whose cycles are irregular, still maturing, or for those who haven't started their first period yet, it's beneficial to align seed cycling with the moon phases. This method mimics a regular menstrual cycle, providing a natural rhythm for the body to follow. In this approach, Phase 1 seeds are consumed from the new moon to the full moon, and Phase 2 seeds are consumed from the full moon to the next new moon. This practice helps to establish and regulate their cycles.

Once a teen's menstrual cycle becomes regular and symptoms such as irregular periods, acne, or PMS are reduced, they can transition to seed cycling based on their own menstrual cycle. This adaptive method ensures that teens can benefit from seed cycling regardless of where they are in their hormonal journey, promoting overall health and well-being.

In summary, seed cycling offers a natural, empowering, and educational way for teens to manage their menstrual health. It promotes the idea that food can be a powerful tool in maintaining hormonal balance and overall well-being, providing a positive and proactive alternative to traditional medical interventions.

Chapter 10
Menopause and Seed Cycling

In today's world, menopause is often portrayed with a focus on its physical symptoms, such as hot flushes and weight gain, leading to fear and dread about this natural transition.

Menopause is often seen as an ending, but within the sisterhood, it's viewed as a powerful rite of passage, a second puberty—one that welcomes women into a community of wisdom and resilience. It's a time to reflect on the life you've lived and the knowledge you've gathered, ready to be shared with those coming after you.

Women entering menopause can be seen as embodying the archetype of the wise elder—a figure revered for her accumulated knowledge, experience, and insight. In many indigenous cultures, menopausal women are honoured for their wisdom and esteemed as leaders, mentors, and spiritual guides within their communities.

From a historical perspective, the purpose of menopause extends beyond its physiological changes. It serves as a natural progression in the life cycle, signalling the completion of a woman's reproductive years and the beginning of a new phase characterised by self-discovery and fulfillment. Menopause invites women to embrace the fullness of their being and to celebrate the richness of their life experience.

Rather than viewing menopause as a decline or loss, I hope we can start to view this phase as an opportunity for reflection, self-discovery, and empowerment. By embracing the wisdom gained through years of lived experience, women can step into new roles with confidence and grace, contributing their unique gifts to the world.

Let's create a movement to reclaim the narrative surrounding menopause, shifting away from fear and stigma toward celebration and empowerment.

The Grandmother Hypothesis

The grandparent effect, also referred to as the grandmother hypothesis in evolutionary biology, it suggests that the presence and engagement of grandparents, particularly grandmothers, play a crucial role in human evolution. This phenomenon underscores the significance of extended family support systems and intergenerational support in the survival and reproductive success of descendants. In the context of menopause, the grandmother hypothesis gains relevance as menopausal women, freed from the demands of reproduction, are uniquely positioned to invest time and resources in supporting their offspring and grandchildren, thereby enhancing their overall fitness.

From an evolutionary perspective, the grandparent effect is crucial for several reasons:

> **Increased Care and Provisioning:** Grandparents, especially grandmothers, play a vital role in providing care, support, and resources to their grandchildren. This assistance can range from food provisioning to childcare, allowing parents to allocate their time and energy more efficiently, ultimately enhancing the survival chances of their offspring.
>
> **Knowledge Transfer:** Grandparents possess valuable knowledge and skills acquired over a lifetime, which they pass down to younger generations. This transmission of knowledge, including cultural traditions, hunting techniques, and medicinal practices, contributes to the adaptive success of human societies by ensuring the continuity of beneficial behaviours across generations.
>
> **Social Cohesion:** The presence of grandparents fosters social cohesion and family bonds within communities. By maintaining

close relationships with their grandchildren and other family members, grandparents strengthen social networks, promote cooperation, and enhance group cohesion, all of which are advantageous for survival and collective well-being.

Life History Theory: In terms of life history theory, the grandparent effect represents a trade-off between investing resources in offspring and investing in one's own survival and reproduction. Grandparents who invest in the care of their grandchildren may forego opportunities for additional offspring of their own but enhance the reproductive success of their existing descendants, thereby perpetuating their genes through indirect means.

Longevity and Kin Selection: The evolution of longevity in humans, particularly post-reproductive lifespan in women, has been linked to the benefits of grand mothering. By extending their lifespan beyond their reproductive years, grandmothers can continue to provide support and guidance to their grandchildren, thus enhancing their inclusive fitness and increasing the likelihood of their genetic legacy being passed on to future generations.

Overall, the grandparent effect illustrates the importance of cooperative breeding and intergenerational cooperation in human evolutionary history. By facilitating resource transfer, knowledge transmission, and social cohesion, grandparents contribute to the adaptive success of families and communities, ultimately shaping the trajectory of human evolution.

My own experiences with my grandparents have been deeply influential, shaping my understanding of family, resilience, and the interconnectedness of generations. Like many, my grandparents served as my teachers, caregivers, and guardians, providing safety and solace during my formative years. I was fortunate to have lived with my grandparents for most of my youth, and their impact on my life has been profound.

At the tender age of five, I experienced the loss of my grandmother from my mum's side, Jelica, who passed away after undergoing a hysterectomy which triggered a brain aneurysm. Reflecting on her untimely death, I can't help but draw parallels to my life's mission today—to share wisdom and empower women to support their hormones naturally. My grandmother's passing was a traumatic event for my family, especially for my mum, who was young and had three small children. Despite her physical absence, I have always felt a strong spiritual connection to my grandmother, sensing her guidance and love throughout my life journey.

Fortunately, I had the privilege of knowing my dad's mother, Vera, until I was twenty years old. She was not only my safety net and caregiver when my mum was working but also my greatest teacher. Vera embodied the essence of sisterhood and the healing power of food as medicine.

Vera's embodiment of sisterhood extended far beyond her immediate family, resonating deeply in her relationships with her own sisters and the community of women who gravitated towards her warmth and kindness. I witnessed this firsthand through the close bond she shared with her sisters, who were not only her family but also her closest confidantes and allies. Their gatherings were filled with laughter, stories, and shared experiences, creating a sense of camaraderie and support that was palpable.

Moreover, Vera's home was a sanctuary for her friends and acquaintances, who would often gather for coffee, cake, and heartfelt conversations. Whether it was in person or over the phone, she offered unwavering support and a listening ear to those in need, while also finding solace and companionship in their presence. Her friendships were built on mutual respect, trust, and reciprocity, with each woman enriching the other's life in meaningful ways.

In addition to fostering connections with others, Vera also imparted her love of food and cooking to me, nurturing my appreciation for fresh ingredients and homemade meals. Her vegetable garden was a labour of love, yielding bountiful harvests of tomatoes that she skilfully transformed into jars of rich, flavourful tomato sauce. The sight of her bustling kitchen, filled with the aroma of freshly baked nut cakes and drying pasta, remains etched in my memory, a testament to her culinary prowess and generosity of spirit.

Through her acts of hospitality, culinary creations, and nurturing presence, Vera exemplified the true essence of sisterhood—a bond forged through shared experiences, mutual support, and a genuine desire to uplift and empower one another. Her legacy lives on in the countless lives she touched and the lessons she imparted, reminding me of the transformative power of connection and community in shaping our lives and nurturing our souls.

Despite facing her own health challenges, including a hysterectomy for hormone issues at a young age, she remained resilient and steadfast in her role as the matriarch of our family.

Now, as my mum enters her grandma era, she continues to offer the same safety and wisdom to my children that my grandmothers provided me. Through their nurturing presence and enduring legacy, my grandparents have instilled in me a profound appreciation for the interconnectedness of past, present, and future generations, reminding me of the importance of passing down wisdom, love, and resilience from one generation to the next.

Understanding Perimenopause and Menopause

Before we dive into strategies for managing this phase, let's understand the basics. Perimenopause marks the transition leading up to menopause, typically beginning in a woman's late 30s or early 40s. It can last from a few years to a decade, during which hormone levels, particularly estrogen and progesterone, fluctuate. Menopause is officially declared after 12 months without a menstrual period.

A Superpower: Needing Fewer Calories

Another fascinating aspect of menopause is the reduced caloric requirements as women age:

> **Efficiency in Caloric Usage:** During menopause, women's metabolism may slow down. Combined with lower caloric needs, this can result in an improved ability to maintain a healthy weight and overall well-being.
>
> **Reduced Risk of Chronic Disease:** Efficiency in resource utilisation during menopause can potentially reduce the risk of

chronic diseases related to aging, such as type 2 diabetes, heart disease, and certain cancers.

Alcohol and Hormonal Changes

The role of alcohol during perimenopause and menopause is significant.

> **Alcohol and Brain Changes:** The hormonal changes during menopause, combined with alcohol consumption, can intensify emotional swings and disrupt sleep patterns. The recalibration of hormones and neurotransmitter fluctuations make women more susceptible to the negative effects of alcohol on mood and sleep.
>
> **Cutting Down on Alcohol:** Reducing or eliminating alcohol can significantly help during this transition, leading to improved sleep, better emotional stability, and a more balanced hormonal profile.

Weight Gain During Menopause

Weight gain during menopause can be a significant fear and source of anxiety for many women. By understanding the underlying reasons and implementing effective strategies, it is possible to mitigate and stop weight gain during this stage of life.

> **Metabolic Changes:** Decreased estrogen levels during menopause can contribute to metabolic changes, including a redistribution of body fat, particularly around the abdomen.
>
> **Muscle Mass Loss:** Aging and hormonal shifts can lead to the loss of muscle mass, which lowers the metabolic rate and makes weight gain more likely. Muscle mass naturally declines with age, and the hormonal changes of menopause can accelerate this process, making it more challenging to maintain a healthy weight.
>
> **Excess Estrogen and EDCs:** Exposure to endocrine-disrupting chemicals (EDCs) and excess estrogen can also contribute to weight gain, particularly around the stomach. EDCs, found in various everyday products, can interfere with hormonal balance, leading to increased fat storage and metabolic

disruptions. Managing exposure to these chemicals and supporting hormonal health can be crucial in addressing weight gain during menopause.

Lifestyle Factors: Changes in activity levels and eating habits, such as increased snacking and decreased physical activity, often accompany menopause. These lifestyle changes can further contribute to weight gain if not managed properly.

Strategies to Mitigate or Reduce Weight Gain During Menopause

Regular Exercise: Prioritise strength training exercises to maintain muscle mass and boost metabolism. Incorporating strength training into your routine is essential for preserving muscle mass, which can decline with age and hormonal changes during menopause. Research suggests that strength training can help manage weight and improve body composition, making it an important component of a menopause weight management plan.

Healthy Diet: Focus on a balanced diet rich in fruits, vegetables, proteins, fibre and natural fats. Reducing the intake of processed foods and refined sugars can help manage weight more effectively.

Mindful Eating: Pay attention to hunger and fullness cues to avoid overeating. Eating mindfully can help prevent unnecessary snacking and promote healthier food choices.

Stress Management: High stress levels can lead to weight gain, particularly around the abdomen. Practices like yoga, EFT, meditation, and deep-breathing exercises can help manage stress and its impact on weight.

Adequate Sleep: Ensure you get enough restful sleep, as poor sleep can disrupt metabolism and increase cravings for unhealthy foods. Aim for 7-9 hours of sleep per night.

Spend Time Outdoors: Spend time outdoors in nature to benefit from its healing and grounding properties. Connecting with nature has been shown to reduce stress, improve mood, and enhance overall well-being. The calming effects of nature can be particularly beneficial during menopause, helping to alleviate symptoms such as anxiety and mood swings.

Cultivate Self-acceptance: The emotional aspect of weight management is significant, as there is often pressure to maintain a certain weight, a common internalised stigma that is deeply ingrained in society. Finding self-acceptance can liberate you from these pressures and support a healthier relationship with your body. Consider working with a practitioner, such as an EFT Tapping Practitioner, to explore techniques for promoting self-acceptance and emotional well-being during menopause.

By understanding the reasons behind menopausal weight gain and adopting a proactive approach, we can navigate this transition more smoothly.

Seed Cycling for Menopause Research

Although formal studies on seed cycling for perimenopausal and menopausal symptoms are still emerging, promising results are being seen through case studies and customer experiences. Many women have reported improvements in symptoms such as hot flushes, mood swings, and sleep disturbances, highlighting seed cycling as a potential natural strategy for managing menopause.

Research on individual seeds used in seed cycling supports their benefits for hormone health during menopause:

Sesame Seeds: A study on postmenopausal women consuming 50g of sesame seeds daily for 5 weeks demonstrated a significant decrease in dehydroepiandrosterone sulfate (DHEAS) levels by 18%, alongside a 15% increase in sex hormone-binding globulin (SHBG) levels, helping to regulate estrogen levels and promote hormonal balance.

Flaxseeds: Numerous studies have linked flaxseeds to improved estrogen levels, better hormone metabolism, and reduced menopausal symptoms, such as hot flushes and vaginal dryness, contributing to overall quality of life during menopause.

Pumpkin Seeds: Rich in magnesium and zinc, pumpkin seeds support hormone balance by alleviating common menopausal symptoms like sleep disturbances and mood swings, through the regulation of progesterone production and stress response.

Sunflower Seeds: Containing high levels of Vitamin E and selenium, sunflower seeds aid estrogen detoxification, reduce oxidative stress, and support thyroid health—key factors in mitigating hot flushes and promoting emotional well-being during menopause.

While more research is needed on seed cycling itself, the scientific findings on individual seeds suggest significant potential for natural, dietary support during menopause.

Seed Cycling, Lunar Rhythm, Moon Phases, and Menopause

The moon has long been revered for its mystical influence on our lives, and its cycles are deeply connected to natural rhythms, including hormonal fluctuations in women. In peri- and post-menopause, aligning with the moon's phases can provide a supportive structure for hormone regulation. As explained in previous chapters, seed cycling with the moon phases offers a wonderful way to reconnect with the lunar rhythm during these transitional stages and beyond.

From the new moon to the full moon, consume Phase 1 seeds—flaxseeds and pumpkin seeds. Then, from the full moon back to the new moon, switch to Phase 2 seeds—sesame and sunflower seeds. This practice aligns with the natural rhythms of the body, even during menopause when menstruation no longer occurs.

For detailed instructions on seed cycling with the moon phases, refer to Chapter 8.

I hope you have enjoyed these insights towards embracing the beauty of cyclical living and finding empowerment within the menopause experience.

Chapter 11
Seed Cycling for PCOS and Other Conditions

Polycystic Ovary Syndrome (PCOS) is a complex hormonal disorder affecting millions of women worldwide, characterised by irregular menstrual cycles, hirsutism (excessive hair growth in areas typical for men) and alopecia (hair thinning or loss), along with acne, mood swings, intense cravings, and insulin resistance.

The exact cause of PCOS is not fully understood, but experts suggest it is likely due to a combination of genetic factors, insulin resistance, hormonal imbalances, and chronic low-grade inflammation. Additionally, lifestyle factors such as diet and stress can influence the severity of symptoms and contribute to the disorder.

When it comes to PCOS management, diet and lifestyle can be powerful tools for symptom management and overall hormone balance. Seed cycling is one promising approach. Studies published in January 2021 and June 2023 have highlighted seed cycling's potential role in managing PCOS symptoms, particularly by supporting estrogen and progesterone balance throughout the cycle.

The study titled "The Effect of Seed Cycling on Polycystic Ovary Syndrome: A Pilot Study," published in Food Science *Nutrients* in 2023 investigated the potential benefits of seed cycling for managing PCOS and involved 60 women aged 15-40 years old over the course of three months. Participants were divided into three groups: a control group, a group practicing portion control and taking metformin (a pharmaceutical drug), and a group practicing portion control while incorporating seed cycling into their diets.

The findings from the research showed promising results for seed cycling in hormone support and PCOS symptom management including:

> **Weight Management:** The group that used seed cycling and portion control experienced a reduction in overall body weight. This is particularly noteworthy for individuals with PCOS, as weight management is often a key aspect of their treatment.
>
> **Hormonal Balance:** In individuals with PCOS, who often have elevated Follicle-Stimulating Hormone (FSH), a decrease in FSH was observed in the group following seed cycling and portion control.
>
> **Cyst Degeneration:** This study referenced the 2021 *Nutraceutical Intervention of Seeds* review, which reported that remarkably, 36% of participants in the seed cycling group experienced complete cyst degeneration, meaning their ovarian cysts either significantly improved or disappeared entirely. In contrast, the control group saw an increase in the number of cysts.
>
> **Luteinizing Hormone (LH) Reduction:** LH levels, another important hormone in the context of PCOS, showed a significant reduction in the seed cycling and portion-controlled group, surpassing the effects of metformin.
>
> **Thyroid-Stimulating Hormone (TSH):** While there was a slight reduction in TSH, it's important to note that this hormone plays a role in overall hormone balance, and even a slight reduction can be beneficial.
>
> **Prolactin Reduction:** Prolactin levels also decreased significantly (by 2%) in the seed cycling and portion-controlled group.

As you can see this study provides some great insights into the benefits of seed cycling for PCOS management, though there are notable limitations to consider:

Seed Cycling for PCOS

Limitations:

- **Limited Dietary Context**: Seed cycling was introduced alongside a portion-controlled diet, but no baseline data on participants' diets before the intervention was available. Without knowing pre-existing dietary habits, it's challenging to isolate the effects of seed cycling alone.

- **Nutritional Deficiency in Calorie Count**: The diet's low calorie intake (around 1500 calories) may not have been adequate for all adult participants, potentially influencing the study's outcomes. A more balanced, sustainable calorie intake could yield even more positive results when paired with seed cycling.

- **Lack of Specific PCOS Typing**: The study did not differentiate among the four PCOS subtypes—post-pill, inflammatory, insulin-resistant, and adrenal. Future research could refine insights by examining how seed cycling impacts each PCOS subtype uniquely.

- **Insufficient Biomarker Analysis**: Additional testing for insulin, androgens, and other hormonal markers could provide a clearer picture of how seed cycling affects specific PCOS-related mechanisms.

Positive Findings:

- **Promising Alternative to Medication**: Seed cycling showed potential benefits comparable to, or even exceeding, the effects of metformin for PCOS symptom management, which is a significant finding for those looking to manage PCOS naturally.

- **Objective Research Context**: With no external funding or grants, the study's findings appear more objective and add credibility to its support for seed cycling as a natural approach to PCOS management.

- **Potential for Hormonal Balance and Cyst Reduction**: The study highlights how seed cycling may support hormonal regulation and reduce cyst formation, suggesting a promising complementary strategy for women with PCOS.

Conclusion: This research opens the door for seed cycling as a natural addition to PCOS management. Incorporating seeds into the diet could positively influence hormonal balance and potentially reduce symptoms. Future studies with a broader dietary perspective, more inclusive calorie levels, and PCOS subtype-specific analysis could provide more targeted insights into this promising approach.

As a result of these findings, there has been newfound interest from General Practitioners (GPs), Universities, and other specialists in seed cycling as an adjunctive therapy for hormone imbalances and PCOS. Since the publication of this study, The Seed Cycle™ has trained numerous GPs and clinics across Australia in seed cycling principles, receiving a warm reception from medical professionals. Recently, The Seed Cycle™ also presented at Torrens University on seed cycling and its study-backed benefits as part of their "Food as Medicine" curriculum, an exciting step forward in educating future health practitioners on integrative approaches to hormonal health

Other research for the individual seeds and PCOS

It has been well documented that the nutraceutical elements present in the seeds can greatly balance the levels of hormones and even reduce weight.

Studies have shown that including flaxseeds can decrease androgen levels in women with PCOS, which can cause excess hair growth and acne, plus improve the cyclical breast tenderness that affects many women before their period.

A 2015 study found regular ingestion of flax seeds over three months caused a significant reduction in the number of ovarian cysts, as well as the size of the ovaries in women with PCOS.

As always, if you have PCOS or any other health condition, it's important to consult with a healthcare professional to create a tailored plan that suits your specific needs and goals.

Seed Cycling for Insulin Sensitivity

Keeping your blood sugar at an optimal level can be difficult for some women due to decreased insulin sensitivity. That means that your cells are less sensitive to insulin, the hormone that helps bring nutrients into the cell and keep blood sugar stable.

Diet and exercise can play an essential role in blood sugar balance. According to a 2020 study, regular flaxseed supplementation for 12 weeks was associated with increased insulin sensitivity and weight loss with patients with PCOS due to the combination of hormone imbalance, insulin resistance and inflammation.

Additionally, the 2021 study found that phytoestrogens in flaxseed bind to 17- beta-estradiol receptors, which may have anti-diabetic effects. This same study noted that both pumpkin seed and flax seed are rich in Omega-3 fatty acids that support cholesterol and insulin sensitivity.

Seed Cycling for Chronic Inflammation

Chronic inflammation is a long-term immune response that can lead to health issues, including hormonal imbalances, cardiovascular diseases, and certain cancers. Unlike acute inflammation, which aids healing, chronic inflammation often arises from lifestyle factors like poor diet, stress, and toxins, disrupting cellular function and increasing oxidative stress.

Research supports that regular seed cycling provides a balanced intake of anti-inflammatory Omega-3 fatty acids, antioxidants, lignans, and minerals, all of which help reduce chronic inflammation and support hormonal balance.

Omega-3 Fatty Acids and Anti-Inflammatory Benefits Seeds rich in Omega-3s, such as flaxseed and pumpkin seeds, help lower inflammatory markers like C-reactive protein (CRP) and interleukin-6 (IL-6). Omega-3s are known to suppress pro-inflammatory molecules, effectively reducing inflammation.

Seed Cycling for Endometriosis

Although there are currently no specific studies on seed cycling for endometriosis, we have heard notable improvements from customers experiencing endometriosis-related symptoms, such as acne, irregular periods, and period pain. These improvements are likely due to the anti-inflammatory properties and hormonal-balancing effects of the seeds used in seed cycling. The nutrients in the seeds may contribute to reduced inflammation and better hormonal regulation, which can help alleviate some symptoms of endometriosis. We remain hopeful that future research will confirm seed cycling as a promising complementary therapy for managing endometriosis.

Seed Cycling for Adenomyosis Support

Adenomyosis, a condition where the tissue that lines the uterus grows into the muscular wall of the uterus, often leads to painful and heavy periods. Seed cycling may offer support for individuals with adenomyosis by promoting hormonal balance and reducing inflammation. Through the targeted consumption of seeds rich in essential fatty acids and phytoestrogens, individuals may experience symptom relief. Research on dietary interventions suggests that omega-3 fatty acids and antioxidants can positively impact uterine health and alleviate symptoms associated with adenomyosis. Although there are currently no specific studies on seed cycling for adenomyosis, we have observed promising improvements in related symptoms, such as irregular periods, among individuals incorporating seed cycling into their diet.

Seed Cycling for Fibroid Management

Fibroids, benign tumours that develop in the uterus, can cause symptoms such as heavy menstrual bleeding, pelvic pain, and reproductive issues. Seed cycling might offer potential benefits for managing fibroids by targeting hormonal imbalances and supporting overall uterine health. Seeds with anti-inflammatory and hormone-regulating properties, such as flaxseeds and pumpkin seeds, could help alleviate symptoms and potentially influence fibroid growth. While there is currently no specific research on the effectiveness of seed cycling for fibroid management, studies on dietary interventions and their impact on uterine health suggest that incorporating nutrient-rich seeds may be beneficial. For example, research on dietary fiber and anti-inflammatory diets highlights their potential role in managing fibroid symptoms. We remain hopeful that future research will further explore and validate seed cycling as a complementary therapy for fibroid management.

Seed Cycling for Thyroid Health

Thyroid conditions, such as hypothyroidism and Hashimoto's thyroiditis, can significantly impact hormone levels and overall well-being. Seed cycling may offer support for individuals with thyroid disorders by providing essential nutrients and promoting hormonal balance. Seeds rich in selenium, zinc, and iodine, such as pumpkin and sunflower seeds, can help support thyroid function and reduce inflammation. By incorporating seed cycling into their routine, individuals with thyroid conditions may experience improved energy levels, better metabolism, and enhanced thyroid hormone production.

Conclusion

While the research on seed cycling for various health conditions is still evolving, the evidence suggests that it holds promise as a natural approach to hormone balance and overall wellness. From managing PCOS and insulin sensitivity to reducing chronic inflammation and supporting reproductive health, seed cycling offers a holistic way to address hormonal imbalances and alleviate symptoms. While it may not be a magic bullet or quick fix, seed cycling can be a valuable addition to comprehensive treatment plans for hormonal conditions. Seed cycling may be the missing puzzle piece you've been searching for on your health journey. If you have or suspect you have any of the conditions listed above it is essential to consult with your healthcare provider.

Chapter 12
Seed Cycling Recipes

Now for one of my favourite parts—I'm sharing with you some of my favourite seed cycling recipes. But first, let's talk about spending time in our kitchens, cooking and baking using real, whole food ingredients—a practice I hold dear not only for its health benefits but also for the meditative and restorative experience it offers. Cooking our meals, even if not every single one, can transform our relationship with food, making it a source of nourishment for both body and soul. The next time you are cooking I invite you to notice how the rhythmic chopping, stirring, and blending, can be incredibly calming and grounding.

For me, seed cycling isn't just about hormone *support*; it's also about establishing a daily ritual that reconnects me with cooking and preparing my meals and considering where I will include an addition of seeds, a meaningful part of my routine.

The Importance of Cooking Our Meals in our Modern World

Cooking at home allows us to be mindful of the ingredients we use, ensuring that our meals are rich in nutrients and free from harmful additives. When we cook, we connect with our food in a way that's impossible with pre-packaged meals or takeaway. The kitchen can become a sanctuary, a place where we can slow down and engage our senses - a mindful experience that grounds us in the present moment.

When we cook with love and intention, it's as if we are infusing our meals with an extra layer of care and nourishment. While it may not be scientifically proven, many of us have experienced the difference in taste between a meal made with genuine affection and one prepared hurriedly out of obligation. There is something almost magical about a dish made with love; it seems to carry a warmth and satisfaction that transcends mere ingredients and technique. The power and love for food and cooking has been passed down through generations, and it's a sentiment shared by many cultures around the world. When we take the time to be present, to enjoy the process, and to cook with a positive mindset, our food often turns out better, not just in flavour but in the joy, it brings to those who share in the meal.

Flexible Recipes for Seed Cycling and Hormone Health

These recipes have been created to be flexible – I encourage you to use what you have in your pantry, fridge and garden. Feel free to make swaps for intolerances and preferences; for example, if a recipe calls for coconut oil but you can't tolerate it, swap it out for ghee or olive oil. You'll notice I use only real food ingredients and, where possible, organic, as this is important, particularly for hormone health. In terms of sweeteners, I prefer real food sweeteners like dates, banana, honey, rice malt syrup, and rapadura sugar. Rapadura sugar and green leaf stevia are my sugars of choice for The Seed Cycle™ Bake Mixes and Seed Cycling + Protein Mixes products as they are unrefined and have nutrients such as iron, calcium, magnesium, and potassium.

You will also notice there is no calorie count on my recipes, this is because I choose to focus on nutrients over calories. The history of calories is rooted in the early 20th century when the calorie was introduced as a measure of energy. However, as Dr. Libby Weaver explains in her book *The Calorie Fallacy*, not all calories are created equal. The quality of the food, the nutrients it provides, and how it interacts with our bodies are far more important than just the caloric content. Counting calories can often lead to an unhealthy focus on quantity over quality, missing the bigger picture of overall well-being.

Finally, I aim to ensure that each recipe delivers the optimal therapeutic dosage for seed cycling when portioned out. This approach not only supports your hormonal health but also aligns with the goal of making your meals and snacks both healing and enjoyable, thereby enhancing the overall therapeutic benefits of the food you consume.

I hope I have inspired you to cook with love and care, using these flexible and nutrient-rich recipes. Enjoy these recipes and experience the profound benefits that seed cycling and cooking can bring to you and your families health.

Hormone Helper Seed Cycle Snaps

This Seed Cycle Snaps recipe provides you with your required daily dose when following your seed cycling practice. These snaps are not only delicious and easy to make, but they also remind me of the sesame seed snaps I used to enjoy as a kid. Be sure to bake them until crispy on a low heat and store in the fridge for freshness.

Makes 14 pieces | Prep Time: 15 minutes

Ingredients

1 container of The Seed Cycle™ Phase 1 or 2

1/2 cup almond meal

1/3 cup rice malt syrup or honey

1/4 cup coconut oil, melted

Pinch of salt

Quality chocolate, melted for topping

Method

Preheat Oven:

Preheat oven to 180 degrees Celsius (350 degrees Fahrenheit).

Combine Ingredients:

In a medium bowl, combine all ingredients and mix well.

Spread Mixture:

Spread the mixture on a lined baking tray.

Place a second piece of baking paper on top of the mixture and spread with a rolling pin or your fingers until the mixture is about 1/2 cm thick.

Bake:

Bake for 10 minutes or until golden and crispy.

Seed Cycling Recipes

Cool and Top:

Once cooled, drizzle with melted chocolate and place in the fridge to set.

Cut and Store:

Cut Seed Snaps into 14 pieces and store in the fridge.

Consume 1 piece each day for Phase 2 of seed cycling.

Enjoy these tasty and nutritious snaps as part of your seed cycling routine to support natural hormone balance!

Seed Cycle + Protein Smoothie Recipes

Smoothies for seed cycling are a quick and convenient way to create a nutrient-dense, balanced meal while ensuring you get your daily dose of The Seed Cycle™. This smoothie is perfect for a busy morning or a refreshing snack.

The Seed Cycle™+ Protein mix includes Inca Inchi and Hemp protein, which provide essential amino acids, Omega-3 fatty acids, and a range of vitamins and minerals to support overall health. Additionally, the mix includes Camu Camu, a superfood rich in Vitamin C and antioxidants, enhancing the nutritional profile of this smoothie.

Makes 1 serving | Prep Time: 5 minutes

Ingredients

1 tablespoon chia seeds

1 cup unsweetened almond milk, coconut water, or milk of choice

1 – 1/2 cups berries

1 tablespoon nut butter

2 scoops seed cycling + protein mix (Phase 1 or 2)

Method

Bloom Chia Seeds:

Pour almond milk and chia seeds into a blender and let sit for 5-10 minutes to allow the chia seeds to bloom.

Add Remaining Ingredients:

Add the remaining ingredients into the blender.

Blend:

Blend until smooth or to your preferred consistency.

Enjoy this delicious and nutritious smoothie as part of your seed cycling routine to support natural hormone balance!

Seed Cycling Recipes

Seed Cycle Harmony Bliss Balls

Crafted to harmonise hormones and tantalise taste buds. Packed with Medjool dates for sweetness and fibre, plus raw cacao for antioxidants, they offer a delicious solution for hormonal health.

Makes 14 servings | Prep Time: 10 minutes

Ingredients

2 tablespoons organic nut butter

8 Medjool dates

3 tablespoons rice malt syrup (optional)

2 tablespoons raw cacao

A pinch of sea salt

2 tablespoons boiling water

1 container of The Seed Cycle™ Phase 1 or 2

Desiccated coconut or raw buckwheat for coating

Method

Blend Ingredients:

Place all the ingredients into a food processor and blend for approximately 3-5 minutes until the mixture comes together.

Roll into Balls:

With wet hands, roll the mixture into balls. Form 14 larger balls or 28 smaller balls to ensure the correct seed dosage.

Adjust Consistency:

If the mixture feels dry, add a little extra water.

Coat and Store:

Roll the balls in desiccated coconut or raw buckwheat. Refrigerate or freeze in an airtight container.

Seed + Oat Salmon Nourish Bowl Recipe

This delicious and nutritious recipe is a collaboration between The Seed Cycle™ and Remedy Kitchen, where we believe in the power of nourishing and wholesome meals to fuel your body and support your hormones.

Serves: 4 | Prep Time: 20 minutes | Cook Time: 10 minutes

Ingredients

4 x salmon steaks, skin off and cut into inch cubes

2 tablespoons of Superb Seasoning Mix

1 cup of cooked brown rice

1 large avocado

1 large cucumber

1 cup of tinned edamame

10 radishes

1 bag of mixed lettuce leaves

Shallots

1 lime

Extra virgin olive oil (EVOO)

Glaze:

4 tablespoons of sesame oil

4 tablespoons of honey

3 tablespoons of tamari

2 teaspoons of finely grated fresh ginger

4 scoops of Seed Cycle

Seed Cycling Recipes

Method

Cook the Rice:

Cook the rice according to the packet instructions.

Prepare the Glaze:

Combine all glaze ingredients and set aside.

Prepare the Salad:

Wash the lettuce, cucumber, radishes, shallots, and edamame. Chop to your liking.

Cook the Salmon:

Cut the salmon into inch cubes and sprinkle with the superb seasoning mix.

Spray your pan with olive oil and cook each side of the salmon cubes for 4-5 minutes.

Turn off the heat before adding the glaze. Toss to evenly cover all the salmon.

Assemble the Bowl:

You can either make individual bowls or serve on a platter.

Start with the lettuce, layer all the ingredients, and finally place the salmon, avocado, shallots, and a squeeze of fresh lime on top.

Phase 1 Vegan Seed Cycle Brownie Bites Recipe

These Vegan Seed Cycle Brownie Bites are perfect for the follicular phase of your menstrual cycle. Packed with nutrients and easy to make, they provide a delicious and healthy snack to support your hormonal health.

Serves: 28 bites | Prep Time: 10 minutes | Cook Time: 15 minutes

Ingredients

1 packet of The Seed Cycle™ Brownie Mix

1/2 cup melted coconut oil

1/2 cup pitted dates

1/4 cup hot filtered water

Method

Soak the Dates:

Soak the dates in hot water for 10-15 minutes to soften.

Prepare the Date Mixture:

Add the soaked dates and the water they were soaking in into a food processor and blend until smooth.

Make the Dough:

Add The Seed Cycle™ Brownie Mix and melted coconut oil to the food processor. Pulse the mixture until it forms a sticky dough.

Form the Brownie Bites:

Roll the dough into 28 small balls. Roll each ball in shredded coconut or raw cacao powder.

Chill and Serve:

Refrigerate the brownie bites for at least 30 minutes before serving. Enjoy 2 Brownie Bites each day as a healthy and delicious snack during the first half of your menstrual cycle.

Seed Cycling Recipes

Store:

Store in the fridge or freezer for optimal freshness.

Seed Cycling Phase 2 Chocolate Raspberry Bars

Indulge in these delicious and healthy Chocolate Raspberry Bars, perfect for the second phase of your menstrual cycle. Easy to make and packed with nutritious ingredients, these bars are a delightful way to support your hormonal health.

Serves: 14 bars | Prep Time: 20 minutes | Cook Time: 30 minutes

Ingredients

1 pack The Seed Cycle™ Biscuit Mix

1/2 cup melted coconut oil

1/2 cup pitted dates

1/4 cup hot filtered water

2 cups quality chocolate, melted (we love Alter Ego Hazelnut Chocolate)

1/2 cup raw buckwheat (optional)

1/3 cup raspberry jam or crushed frozen raspberries

27.5 x 3.5 cm baking tray and baking paper

Method

Soak the Dates:

Soak the dates in hot water for 10-15 minutes to soften.

Prepare the Date Mixture:

Add the soaked dates and the water they were soaking in into a food processor and blend until smooth.

Make the Dough:

Add The Seed Cycle™ Biscuit Mix and melted coconut oil to the food processor. Pulse the mixture until it forms a sticky dough.

Seed Cycling Recipes

Form the Base Layer:

Split the mixture in half and press half the mixture evenly onto a lined baking tray, creating a layer approximately 1.5 cm thick.

Add the Raspberry Layer:

Top the base layer with raspberry jam and sprinkle with raw buckwheat if using. Freeze for 15 minutes.

Form the Top Layer:

Remove the tray from the freezer and add the rest of the dough, spreading it evenly over the raspberry layer. Freeze again for 15-30 minutes.

Coat in Chocolate:

Once set, cut the mixture into 14 bars and coat each bar in melted chocolate. Freeze the bars on a lined baking tray until the chocolate has set.

Store and Enjoy:

Store the bars in a glass container in the freezer. Enjoy one Chocolate Raspberry Bar each day as a healthy and delicious snack during the second half of your menstrual cycle.

Seed Cycle Crackers Recipe

These Seed Cycle Crackers are a nutritious and delicious way to get your daily dose of Phase 1 or Phase 2 seeds. Perfect as a snack or accompaniment to your meals, these crackers are easy to make and customisable to suit your taste.

Serves: 15 crackers | Prep Time: 10 minutes | Cook Time: 25 minutes

Ingredients

5 scoops Seed Cycle Phase 1 or Phase 2

2 tablespoons psyllium husk

1/4 teaspoon sea salt

1 teaspoon spices of your choice (paprika, turmeric, onion, and nutmeg are great)

1/2 cup water

Sea salt flakes and pumpkin seeds for topping (optional)

Method

Preheat the Oven:

Preheat the oven to 160°C.

Mix Dry Ingredients:

In a medium bowl, combine all the dry ingredients.

Add Water:

Add water to the bowl and stir until the mixture becomes a thick dough.

Roll Out Dough:

Roll the dough between two sheets of baking paper until it is 1/2 cm thick.

Seed Cycling Recipes

Prepare for Baking:

Remove the top sheet of parchment paper and add toppings if desired. Use a knife to score the dough into 15 equal squares.

Bake:

Bake for 20-25 minutes or until the crackers are golden brown.

Serve:

Break the crackers apart along the scored lines. Enjoy 3 crackers each day to fulfill your seed cycle daily dose.

Choc Rice Puffs Recipe

These Choc Rice Puffs are a delightful way to get your daily dose of Phase 1 seeds from The Seed Cycle™. With a combination of crunchy puffed rice and rich chocolate, these treats are both nutritious and satisfying.

Serves: 28 patty cakes or 14 pieces | Prep Time: 10 minutes | Chill Time: 15 minutes

Ingredients

1 container of Seed Cycle Phase 1

2 cups organic puffed rice

1/3 cup extra virgin coconut oil

1/3 cup raw cacao powder

1/3 cup rice malt syrup

Pinch of salt

Method

Melt Ingredients:

Melt coconut oil, rice malt syrup, and cacao melts on the stove or in the microwave. Mix until smooth.

Combine Ingredients:

Mix through puffed rice, Seed Cycle Phase 1, and salt.

Prepare for Setting:

Place the mixture into 28 lined muffin tins or a pan. Use the back of a spoon or a piece of baking paper and a rolling pin to press the mixture firmly into place.

Chill:

Place in the freezer for 10-15 minutes

Seed Cycling Recipes

Serve:

Store in an airtight container in the fridge. Enjoy 2 patty cakes or 1 piece each day for your daily dose of seed cycling.

Seed Cycle Yoghurt Bowl Recipe

Elevate your breakfast or snack with this nutritious and delicious Seed Cycle Yoghurt Bowl. Packed with fresh flavours and supportive nutrients, it's an easy and delightful way to incorporate seed cycling into your routine.

Serves: 1 | Prep Time: 5 minutes

Ingredients

1/2 to 1 cup of your favourite yoghurt (we recommend coconut yoghurt for a creamy, dairy-free option)

A handful of fresh or frozen berries (such as blueberries, raspberries, or strawberries)

1 serving of Seed Cycle Phase 1 or Phase 2 (depending on your cycle phase) or Seed Cycle + Protein mix for extra protein

Optional toppings:

Crumbled Seed Cycle Biscuits

Sliced banana

Chia seeds

Other seasonal fruits

Nuts (like almonds or walnuts)

A drizzle of honey or maple syrup for added sweetness

Method

Prepare the Base:

Start with 1/2 to 1 cup of your favourite yoghurt in a bowl.

Add Fruit:

Add a handful of fresh or frozen berries for a burst of flavour and extra nutrients.

Seed Cycling Recipes

Mix in Seeds:

Scoop in one serving of Seed Cycle Phase 1 or Phase 2, or use The Seed Cycle™ + Protein mix for an extra protein boost. Mix well to combine.

Top It Off:

Enhance your bowl with optional toppings such as crumbled Seed Cycle Biscuits, sliced banana, chia seeds, flaxseeds, nuts, and a drizzle of honey or maple syrup.

Enjoy:

Mix well and savour the delicious flavours and health benefits!

Goodbye PMS Avocado Choc Mousse Recipe

Indulge in this creamy, nutrient-packed Avocado Choc Mousse. Perfect as a delicious and healthy dessert, it's infused with superfoods and designed to support your hormonal balance.

Serves: 2 | Prep Time: 10 minutes | Chill Time: 30 minutes

Ingredients

2 ripe avocados

1/3 cup raw cacao powder

1 tsp maca powder

1-2 tsp collagen powder

1/2 - 1 cup rice malt syrup (depending on desired sweetness)

A pinch of salt

1-2 tablespoons almond milk

1 scoop Seed Cycle Phase 2

Method

Prepare the Avocados:

Cut open the avocados and remove the pits. Scoop out the flesh and place it into a blender or food processor.

Add Dry Ingredients:

Add the cacao powder, maca powder, collagen powder, rice malt syrup, and a pinch of salt. Blend until smooth and creamy.

Blend to Perfection:

Gradually add the almond milk, one tablespoon at a time, and blend until the mixture has a smooth and mousse-like consistency.

Adjust Sweetness:

Taste the mousse and adjust the sweetness as needed by adding more rice malt syrup.

Chill and Serve:

Spoon the mousse into small cups and chill in the fridge for at least 30 minutes before serving.

Garnish:

Serve with fresh berries, chopped nuts, and an extra sprinkle of Seed Cycle Phase 2 for added texture and nutrients.

Estrogen Detox Carrot & Lentil Salad Recipe

This vibrant Carrot & Lentil Salad is packed with nutrients and flavours, perfect for a refreshing and wholesome meal. Incorporate Seed Cycle Phase 1 or 2 to support your hormonal balance.

Serves: 4 | Prep Time: 20 minutes | Cook Time: 30 minutes

Ingredients

4 cups grated carrots

2 cups dried lentils, soaked & cooked (or canned lentils)

1 cup medjool dates, pitted and chopped

1 small red onion, finely chopped

5 spring onions, chopped

Dressing:

1/4 cup extra virgin olive oil

Zest and juice of two limes

1 teaspoon ground cumin

1/2 teaspoon fresh or ground grated nutmeg

1/2 teaspoon turmeric

Pinch of chili flakes

Himalayan salt and pepper to taste

To Serve:

1/2 cup roasted pistachios

1 cup crumbled goat's feta

Seed Cycle Phase 1 or 2

Method

Prepare the Salad:

In a large bowl, combine the grated carrots, lentils, chopped dates, red onion, and spring onions.

Make the Dressing:

In a separate bowl, whisk together the olive oil, lime zest and juice, ground cumin, nutmeg, turmeric, chili flakes, salt, and pepper until well combined.

Dress the Salad:

Pour the dressing over the carrot and lentil mixture and toss to coat evenly.

Serve and Garnish:

Garnish the salad with roasted pistachios, crumbled goat's feta, and a sprinkle of Seed Cycle Phase 1 or 2.

Hormone Support Green Banana Flour Pancakes

These Green Banana Flour Pancakes are not only delicious but also support your hormonal balance with the inclusion of Seed Cycle Phase 2. Perfect for a nourishing breakfast or snack!

Green banana flour is rich in resistant starch, which supports gut health, aids in digestion, and helps regulate blood sugar levels.

Serves: 2 | Prep Time: 10 minutes | Cook Time: 10 minutes

Ingredients

1/2 cup banana flour

1/3 cup buckwheat flour or almond meal

1/2 teaspoon baking powder

2 free range eggs

1 tablespoon rice malt syrup or monk fruit sugar (low carb option)

1/2 teaspoon organic vanilla extract

1/3 cup milk of choice

Coconut oil, for frying

Blueberries or chocolate chips (optional)

Topping Suggestions:

Berries, butter, rice malt syrup & cinnamon

Yoghurt and Seed Cycle Phase 2

Method

Prepare the Batter:

In a medium bowl, combine the banana flour, buckwheat flour or almond meal, and baking powder.

Add the eggs, rice malt syrup or monk fruit sugar, vanilla extract, and milk. Mix until well combined.

Seed Cycling Recipes

Heat the Pan:

Heat a small amount of coconut oil in a pan over low to medium heat. (Note: Banana flour should not be heated at high temperatures.)

Cook the Pancakes:

Pour small amounts of batter into the pan to make small pancakes.

Cook until bubbles form on the surface, then flip and cook until golden brown on both sides.

Serve:

Serve with 1 scoop of Seed Cycle Phase 2 and your choice of toppings such as berries, butter, rice malt syrup & cinnamon, or yoghurt.

Seed Cycle Toast Toppers

Elevate your morning toast with these nutrient-packed Seed Cycle Toast Toppers, perfect for a delicious and hormone-supportive start to your day.

Ingredients

½ - 1 avocado, roughly mashed

2 pieces spelt sourdough bread

Squeeze of lemon juice or sprinkle of sumac powder

1 scoop Phase 1 or 2 The Seed Cycle™

Method

Toast your bread to your desired level of crispiness.

Spread the mashed avocado evenly over the toast.

Sprinkle with lemon juice or sumac powder.

Finish with a scoop of The Seed Cycle™ Phase 1 or 2.

For extra protein and iron, you can spread some hummus or liver pate on your toast before adding the avocado. Enjoy your Seed Cycle Toast Toppers for a delicious and hormone-supportive breakfast!

Seed Cycling Recipes

Seed Cycling Matcha Slice Recipe

The Seed Cycling Matcha Breakfast Slice is a delightful creation by Grace Martin, renowned for her inventive culinary skills. As a co-host on the Unprocessed podcast within the I Quit Sugar series, Grace brings her innovative touch to the world of nutritious and flavourful recipes. I even had the pleasure of joining Grace as a guest on the I Quit Sugar Podcast episode titled "The Hormone Whisperer Reveals The Seed Cycling Secret to Happy Hormones."

Serving Size: 6 slices | Prep Time: 25 minutes | Setting Time: overnight

Ingredients

Crust:

1/2 cup oats

1/2 cup shredded coconut

8 Medjool dates, unpitted (for natural sweetness and binding)

2 tablespoons almond spread (providing creaminess and rich in vitamin E)

3 tablespoons almond milk

6 scoops The Seed Cycle™ Phase 1 or 2 blend

Filling:

1 tablespoon matcha (a superfood loaded with antioxidants)

1 cup raw cashews (for creaminess and healthy fats)

1/4 cup rice malt syrup

1 cup coconut cream (adding a lush, tropical richness)

1 teaspoon vanilla extract

Method

Soften the cashews by boiling them in a saucepan, then let them sit for 15 minutes to become pliable.

While the cashews are softening, soak the Medjool dates in hot water for 10 minutes to soften them as well.

Line a slice tray with baking paper to ensure easy removal.

In a food processor, blend the quick oats, shredded coconut, softened dates, almond spread, almond milk, and The Seed Cycle™ Phase 1 or 2 blend until a sticky, cohesive mixture forms.

Press the crust mixture evenly into the prepared slice tray and place it in the freezer to set while you prepare the filling.

Clean the food processor and blend the soaked cashews, matcha, rice malt syrup, coconut cream, and vanilla extract until smooth and creamy.

Pour the green filling over the set crust, smoothing it out for an even layer.

Return the tray to the freezer and let it set until firm, ideally overnight, to ensure the layers meld together perfectly.

When ready to serve, slice the creation into bars or squares and indulge in a piece of this Seed Cycling Matcha masterpiece.

Acknowledgments

Creating *Seeds of Sisterhood* has been a journey filled with inspiration, joy, and unwavering support from those around me. I would like to extend my heartfelt gratitude to everyone who has played a part in bringing this book to life.

To my first readers and editors, thank you for your invaluable insights and encouragement as I shaped this work. A special thank you to my mother, Mira, and my dear friend Sami, who have not only shared in my vision but have supported me with warmth, wisdom, and honest feedback.

To my mentors and teachers, thank you for guiding me and generously sharing your knowledge. Your wisdom has been a beacon on my path, helping me grow and shape my voice as a writer and storyteller. I am deeply grateful for each lesson, each insight, and every moment of guidance you've provided.

To my husband, whose name isn't mentioned elsewhere in the pages but who has been an invisible yet powerful presence throughout. You have been my greatest champion and have stood by me through every step. From supporting The Seed Cycle™ to taking on the countless everyday tasks that allowed me to focus on my writing, to handling the marketing, and always pushing me to see my own worth—you have been there, unconditionally. Thank you for believing in me, for helping me grow, and for reminding me to value my time.

To each person who contributed to this book, both directly and indirectly, I am grateful for your role in making *Seeds of Sisterhood* a reality. Your support has been the foundation that helped me tell this story. Thank you.

The Seed Cycle™ Resources

Seed Cycle Tracker
https://theseedcycle.au/pages/seed-cycle-tracker

Seed Cycle Recipes
https://theseedcycle.au/blogs/recipes

The Seed Cycle™ Cookbook
https://theseedcycle.au/pages/seed-cycling-for-hormone-balance-cookbook

Hormone Health Challenge
https://theseedcycle.au/pages/hormone-reset-challenge-new

Seed Cycle Directory
https://theseedcycle.au/pages/seed-cycling-directory

Complete Seed Cycling Guide
https://theseedcycle.au/pages/seed-cycling-ebook

Recommendations: Books and Courses

First Moon Circle School. (n.d.). *First Moon Circle School: Menstrual education for girls and their families.* https://firstmooncircleschool.com/

Naturopathic WomanCraft. (n.d.). *The Empowered Puberty Journey: Supporting girls through the transition to womanhood.* https://www.naturopathicwomancraft.com.au/the-empowered-puberty-journey

Brighten, J. (2019). *Beyond the Pill: A 30-Day Program to Balance Your Hormones, Reclaim Your Body, and Reverse the Dangerous Side Effects of the Birth Control Pill.* HarperOne.

Brighten, J. (2020). *The Period Repair Manual: Natural Treatment for Better Hormones and Better Periods.* Lulu Publishing Services.

Vitti, A. (2020). *In the Flow: Unlock Your Hormonal Advantage and Revolutionize Your Life.* HarperOne.

Peach, L. (2019). *Period Queen: Life Hack Your Cycle and Own Your Power All Month Long.* Murdoch Books.

Briden, L. (2017). *The Period Repair Manual: Natural Treatment for Better Hormones and Better Periods.* Hay House Inc.

Pelz, M. (2022). *Fast Like a Girl: A Woman's Guide to Using the Healing Power of Fasting to Burn Fat, Boost Energy, and Balance Hormones.* Hay House Inc.

Hardwicke Collings, J. (n.d.). *Complete Collection: Six Books.* Jane Hardwicke Collings. Retrieved from https://janehardwickecollings.com/product/complete-collection-six-books/

Naturopathic Woman Craft. (n.d.). *Cyclical Recipe Guide.* Retrieved from https://www.naturopathicwomancraft.com.au/product/cyclical-recipe-guide/37?cs=true&cst=custom

Bolen, J.S. (1984). *Goddesses in Everywoman: Powerful Archetypes in Women's Lives*. Harper & Row.

Steph Lowe. Understanding PMS and PMDD Masterclass https://the-natural-nutritionist.teachable.com/p/understanding-pms-pmdd

The Nutrition Academy: https://thenutrition.academy/ use code: *'SEEDCYCLE'* for a special discount.

References

Introduction and Definitions:

"Seeds are nutritional powerhouses:" Better Health Victoria. (n.d.). *Seeds are nutritional powerhouses*. Retrieved October 28, 2024, from https://www.betterhealth.vic.gov.au/health/healthyliving/Nuts-and-seeds

"Movement of the 1960s and 1970s, emphasising unity and collective action among women:" Fiveable. (2024). *The 1970s women's liberation movement*. Retrieved October 18, 2024 from https://library.fiveable.me/key-terms/feminist-art-history/the-1970s-womens-liberation-movement

Transformations in the women's liberation movement in the 1970s:" Dinerstein, A., & Kelsey, A. (Eds.). (2022). *Rethinking feminist activism: Transformations in the women's liberation movement in the 1970s*. Routledge.

Chapter 1: The Medicine Women and Mother Nature

"Healing and the role of women:" Ehrenreich, B., & English, D. (1973). *Witches, Midwives, and Nurses: A History of Women Healers*. Feminist Press.

O'Connor, B. B. (1995). *Healing Traditions: Alternative Medicine and the Health Professions*. University of Pennsylvania Press. Retrieved October 18, 2024 from https://theherbalacademy.com/blog/herbalism-a-history/

"healers were suppressed, destroyed, or intentionally hidden:" Ehrenreich, B., & English, D. (2010). *Witches, midwives, & nurses: A history of women healers*. Feminist Press at the City University of New York

The Herbal Academy. (n.d.). *Herbalism: A History – How Herbalists Of The Past Paved The Way For Today*.

"Witch hunts and persecution:" National Archives. (n.d.). Witch hunts and persecution. Retrieved October 28, 2024, from https://www.nationalarchives.gov.uk/education/resources/early-modern-witch-trials/

"Colonialism and cultural suppression:" Campbell, D., Burgess, C. P., Garnett, S. T., & Wakerman, J. (2011). Potential primary health care savings for chronic disease care associated with Australian Aboriginal involvement in land management. Health Policy, 99(1), 83-89. https://doi.org/10.1016/j.healthpol.2010.07.009

"Cultural borrowing and sharing:" Aboriginal bush medicine in practice:" Ralph-Flint, J. (2001). Cultural borrowing and sharing: Aboriginal bush medicine in practice. Australian Journal of Holistic Nursing, 8(1), 43-46. Retrieved October 18, 2024 from https://healthinfonet.ecu.edu.au/learn/cultural-ways/traditional-healing-and-medicine/

"Medicalisation of healthcare:" Hofmann, B. (2016). Medicalisation and overdiagnosis: What society does to medicine. International Journal of Health Policy and Management, 5(11), 619-622. https://doi.org/10.15171/ijhpm.2016.121

"The Library of Ashurbanipal in ancient Assyria destroyed:" World History Encyclopedia. (n.d.). The Library of Ashurbanipal in ancient Assyria destroyed. Retrieved October 18, 2024 from https://www.worldhistory.org/Library_of_Ashurbanipal/

"Resurgence of interest in traditional healing practices:" Earl, A., & Larkins, S. (2022). Adapting traditional healing values and beliefs into therapeutic cultural environments for health and well-being. International Journal of Environmental Research Research and and Public Health, 19 Public(1), 426. https://doi.org/10.3390/ijerph19010426

"Medicine Women, Agnodice:" A brief history of women in medicine:" Women in Antiquity. (2021). Agnodice: A brief history of women in medicine. Retrieved from https://womeninantiquity.wordpress.com/2021/04/02/agnodice/

"Root cause analysis:" National Center for Biotechnology Information. (2024). Root cause analysis and medical error prevention. Updated

February 12, 2024. Retrieved from
https://www.ncbi.nlm.nih.gov/books/NBK570638/

"Food as medicine:" BMJ. (2020). Food is medicine: Actions to integrate food and nutrition into healthcare. BMJ, 369. https://doi.org/10.1136/bmj.m2482

"Traditional Chinese medicine:" Encyclopedia Britannica, Inc. (n.d.). Traditional Chinese medicine. Retrieved October 28, 2024, from https://www.britannica.com/science/traditional-Chinese-medicine

"A glimpse of Ayurveda – The forgotten history and principles of Indian traditional medicine:" Jaiswal, Y. S., & Williams, L. L. (2017). A glimpse of Ayurveda – The forgotten history and principles of Indian traditional medicine. Journal of Traditional Complementary Medicine, 7(1), 50–53. https://doi.org/10.1016/j.jtcme.2016.02.002

"Indigenous Australians understanding of the therapeutic benefits of local flora:" NATIF. (n.d.). Health benefits of Australian native foods. Retrieved October 28, 2024, from https://natif.com.au/blogs/news/health-benefits-of-australian-native-foods

"Australian native fruits: Potential uses as functional food ingredients:" Richmond, R., Bowyer, M., & Vuong, Q. (n.d.). Australian native fruits: Potential uses as functional food ingredients. School of Environmental and Life Sciences, University of Newcastle.

"The role of functional foods, nutraceuticals, and food supplements in intestinal health:" Nutrients. (2010). The role of functional foods, nutraceuticals, and food supplements in intestinal health. Nutrients, 2(6), 611–625.

"Functional foods are rich sources of micronutrients, antioxidants, and bioactive compounds;" Essa, M. M., Bishir, M., Bhat, A., Chidambaram, S. B., Al-Balushi, B., Hamdan, H., Govindarajan, N., Freidland, R. P., & Qoronfleh, M. W. (2023). Functional foods and their impact on health. *Journal of Food Science and Technology*, 22, Article 9998796. https://pmc.ncbi.nlm.nih.gov/articles/PMC9998796/

A comprehensive review on nutraceuticals: Therapy support and formulation challenges:" Nutrition Research Reviews. (2022). A comprehensive review on nutraceuticals: Therapy support and formulation challenges. Volume 14(21), 4637. Retrieved October 18, 2024 from https://www.ncbi.nlm.nih.gov/pmc/articles/PMC9654660/

"Introduction:" Goldberg, I. (Ed.). (1994). Functional foods. Chapman and Hall.

"Mother Earth, Gaia:" Theoi. (n.d.). Mother Earth, Gaia. Retrieved from https://www.theoi.com/Protogenos/Gaia2.html

Chapter 2: Functional Nutrition, EFT and Our Body's Innate Intelligence

Functional Nutrition: The Nutrition Academy. (n.d.). Retrieved September 24, 2024, from https://thenutrition.academy/

Emotional Freedom Techniques: *Journal of Evidence-Based Integrative Medicine.* (2019). Emotional Freedom Techniques. *Journal of Evidence-Based Integrative Medicine, 24*, Article 2515690X18823691. Published online February 19, 2019. PMCID: PMC6381429. PMID: 30777453.

Cyndi Omeara, Functional Nutrition: Changing Habits. (n.d.). Cyndi O'Meara's Story. Retrieved September 24, 2024, from https://changinghabits.com.au/cyndis-story/

"Emotional Freedom Techniques:" Stapleton, P. (2022). Science of Tapping. Available at: https://www.petastapleton.com/science-of-tapping-2022

"What Is EFT Tapping?:" WebMD. (2021). What Is EFT Tapping? Medically reviewed by Dan Brennan, MD on October 25, 2021. Written by WebMD Editorial Contributors. Retrieved September 24, 2024, from https://www.webmd.com/mental-health/what-is-eft-tapping

The Tapping Solution: Ortner, N. (2013). *The Tapping Solution: A Revolutionary System for Stress-Free Living.* Hay House.

EFT for PTSD: Libretto, S., Hilton, L., Gordon, S., Zhang, W., & Wesch, J. (2015). Clinical report: Effects of Integrative PTSD Treatment in a Military Health Setting. *Energy Psychology*, 7(2).

"**Intuitive Eating Scale–2:**" Tylka, T. L., & Kroon Van Diest, A. M. (2013). The Intuitive Eating Scale–2: Item refinement and psychometric evaluation with college women and men. *Journal of Counseling Psychology, 60*(1), 137-153. https://doi.org/10.1037/a0030893

"**Research indicates that those who practice intuitive eating are less likely to engage in disordered eating behaviours:**" Tribole, E., & Resch, E. (2020). *Intuitive Eating: A Revolutionary Anti-Diet Approach*. St. Martin's Essentials.

Mindful Eating: Albers, S. (2008). *Eat, Drink, and Be Mindful: How to End Your Struggle with Mindless Eating and Start Savoring Food with Intention and Joy*. New Harbinger Publications.

Intuitive Eating and Health Indicators: Van Dyke, N., & Drinkwater, E. J. (2014). Relationships between intuitive eating and health indicators: Literature review. *Public Health Nutrition, 17*(8), 1757-1766. https://doi.org/10.1017/S1368980013002139

Mindfulness-Based Eating Awareness: Kristeller, J. L., & Wolever, R. Q. (2011). Mindfulness-based eating awareness training for treating binge eating disorder: The conceptual foundation. *Eating Disorders, 19*(1), 49-61. https://doi.org/10.1080/10640266.2011.533605

Acceptance and Commitment Therapy: Lillis, J., & Kendra, K. E. (2014). Acceptance and Commitment Therapy for weight self-stigma: A case study. *Cognitive and Behavioral Practice, 21*(2), 281-290. https://doi.org/10.1016/j.cbpra.2013.10.005

Health at Every Size: Provencher, V., & Bégin, C. (2018). Health at Every Size: A Weight-Neutral Approach for Empowerment, Resilience and Transformation. *Journal of Obesity & Eating Disorders, 2*(1), 1-3.

Chapter 3: Endocrine System and Hormone Balance

"Globally, 90% of women will experience at least one symptom of premenstrual syndrome (PMS):" Johns Hopkins Medicine. (n.d.). *Premenstrual Syndrome (PMS) and Premenstrual Dysphoric Disorder (PMDD)*. Retrieved October 30, 2024, from https://www.hopkinsmedicine.org/health/conditions-and-diseases/premenstrual-dysphoric-disorder-pmdd

"Epidemiological and Clinical Characteristics of Premenstrual Syndrome and Premenstrual Dysphoric Disorder." Gao, M., Zhang, W., & Guo, W. (2022). Epidemiological and Clinical Characteristics of Premenstrual Syndrome and Premenstrual Dysphoric Disorder. *Journal of Women's Health*, 31(3), 234-240.

"8-13% of women are diagnosed with polycystic ovarian syndrome (PCOS):" World Health Organization. (2023). *Polycystic Ovary Syndrome (PCOS) Fact Sheet*. Retrieved October 30, 2024, from https://www.who.int/news-room/fact-sheets/detail/polycystic-ovary-syndrome

"Polycystic ovary syndrome:" A complex condition with psychological, reproductive, and metabolic manifestations that impacts on health across the lifespan." Teede, H., Deeks, A., & Moran, L. (2010). Polycystic ovary syndrome: A complex condition with psychological, reproductive, and metabolic manifestations that impacts on health across the lifespan. *BMC Medicine*, 8, 41.

"Endometriosis:" Giudice, L. C. (2010). Endometriosis. *The New England Journal of Medicine*, 362(25), 2389-2398.

Office on Women's Health. (2019). *Endometriosis*. U.S. Department of Health and Human Services. Retrieved October 30, 2024, from https://www.womenshealth.gov/a-z-topics/endometriosis

"The Androgen Excess and PCOS Society criteria for the polycystic ovary syndrome:" The complete task force report." Azziz, R., Carmina, E., Dewailly, D., Diamanti-Kandarakis, E., Escobar-Morreale, H. F., Futterweit, W., ... & Witchel, S. F. (2009). The Androgen Excess and PCOS Society criteria for the polycystic ovary syndrome: The complete task force

report. *Fertility and Sterility*, 91(2), 456-488.
https://doi.org/10.1016/j.fertnstert.2008.06.035

"for men, a hormone imbalance such as low testosterone levels affects around 2.1%:" Araujo, A. B., Esche, G. R., Kupelian, V., O'Donnell, A. B., Travison, T. G., & McKinlay, J. B. (2007). Prevalence of symptomatic androgen deficiency in men. *The Journal of Clinical Endocrinology & Metabolism*, 92(11), 4241–4247.

"Clinical experts in the field validate these findings, affirming the widespread occurrence of hormone-related issues in their female clinics": Gottfried, S. (2013). *The Hormone Cure: Reclaim Balance, Sleep, Sex Drive, and Vitality Naturally with the Gottfried Protocol*. Scribner.

"Period problems have been accepted in society:" United Nations Population Fund. (n.d.). Period shame, misinformation linked to serious human rights concerns. *UNFPA*. Retrieved October 30, 2024, from https://www.unfpa.org/news/period-shame-misinformation-linked-serious-human-rights-concerns

"hormones not only govern the menstrual cycle and reproductive health but also exert profound influences on mood, metabolism, skin health, and bone density:" University Hospitals. (n.d.). Estrogen's effects on the female body. *University Hospitals Health Encyclopedia*. Retrieved October 30, 2024, from https://www.uhhospitals.org/health-information/health-and-wellness-library/article/adult-diseases-and-conditions-v0/estrogens-effects-on-the-female-body

"Situated in the brain, the hypothalamus and pituitary gland serve as command centers:" TeachMePhysiology. (n.d.). Menstrual Cycle - HPG Axis - Stages. *TeachMePhysiology*. Retrieved October 30, 2024, from https://teachmephysiology.com/reproductive-system/development-maturation/menstrual-cycle/

"The documentation and discussion of hormone imbalances in women can be traced back to ancient times:" Oneworld Ayurveda. (n.d.). Ayurveda and Women's Health: A Holistic Approach to Hormonal Balance. *Oneworld Ayurveda*. Retrieved October 30, 2024, from https://oneworldayurveda.com/blog/ayurveda-and-womens-health/

In Traditional Chinese Medicine (TCM), texts dating back thousands of years mention the concept of 'yin' and 'yang': Anonymous. (n.d.). *Huangdi Neijing* [The Yellow Emperor's Inner Canon].

Sharma, R. K., & Dash, B. (2007). *Charaka Samhita*. Chowkhamba Sanskrit Series Office.

Singh, B. (2010). *Sushruta Samhita*. Chaukhamba Surbharati Prakashan.

"In Western medicine, the formal study and documentation of hormone imbalances in women began to emerge during the 19th and early 20th centuries:" Medvei, V. C. (1982). *A History of Endocrinology*. Springer. Retrieved October 30, 2024, from https://link.springer.com/book/10.1007/978-94-009-7304-6

"Despite advances in diagnostic tools and treatments for conditions like polycystic ovary syndrome (PCOS) and endometriosis, many women still feel dissatisfied with the available solutions:" Ebert, M. (2024). Study reveals critical gaps in care for PCOS patients. *Contemporary OB/GYN*. Retrieved October 30, 2024, from https://www.contemporaryobgyn.net/view/study-reveals-critical-gaps-in-care-for-pcos-patients

"Michigan Health System in 2015 found that nearly one in five women who undergo a hysterectomy may not need the procedure:" University of Michigan Health System. (2015). Unnecessary hysterectomies? Nearly 1 in 5 women could have avoided the procedure, study suggests. *University of Michigan Health System News*. Retrieved October 30, 2024, from https://www.uofmhealth.org/news/archive/201501/unnecessary-hysterectomies-nearly-1-5-women-could-have

"There are three primary forms of estrogen, with a fourth form exclusively produced during pregnancy:" Mayo Clinic. (n.d.). Estrogen: What are the different types? *Mayo Clinic*. Retrieved October 30, 2024, from https://www.mayoclinic.org/healthy-lifestyle/womens-health/expert-answers/estrogen/faq-20058439

"Production and actions of estrogens." Gruber, C. J., Tschugguel, W., Schneeberger, C., & Huber, J. C. (2002). Production and actions of estrogens. *The New England Journal of Medicine*, 346(5), 340-352. https://doi.org/10.1056/NEJMra000471

"Produced primarily in the ovaries, progesterone helps prepare the uterine lining for implantation of a fertilized egg during the luteal phase of the menstrual cycle:" Progesterone: Natural Function, Levels & Side Effects. (n.d.). *Cleveland Clinic*. Retrieved October 30, 2024, from https://my.clevelandclinic.org/health/body/24562-progesterone

Neurosteroids:" Schumacher, M., & Baulieu, E.-E. (2005). Neurosteroids: From Definition and Biochemistry to Physiopathologic Function. In *Neurosteroids: A New Regulatory Function in the Nervous System* (pp. 1–25). Springer. Retrieved October 30, 2024, from https://link.springer.com/chapter/10.1007/978-1-59259-693-5_1

"During menopause, testosterone levels, along with estrogen and progesterone, typically decline:" Davison, S. L., Bell, R., Donath, S., Montalto, J. G., & Davis, S. R. (2005). Androgen Levels in Adult Females: Changes with Age, Menopause, and Oophorectomy. *The Journal of Clinical Endocrinology & Metabolism*, 90(7), 3847–3853. Retrieved October 30, 2024, from https://doi.org/10.1210/jc.2005-0212

"Female sex hormones that play important roles in the body:" Merck Manuals. (n.d.). Follicle-stimulating hormone (FSH) levels test. *Merck Manuals*. Retrieved October 30, 2024, from https://www.merckmanuals.com/-/media/Manual/LabTests/FollicleStimulatingHormoneFSHLevelsTest.html

WebMD. (n.d.). Luteinizing hormone (LH) test. *WebMD*. Retrieved October 30, 2024, from https://www.webmd.com/a-to-z-guides/luteinizing-hormone-test

WebMD. (n.d.). Prolactin levels test: High vs. low, normal range. *WebMD*. Retrieved October 30, 2024, from https://www.webmd.com/a-to-z-guides/prolactin-test

SpringerLink. (2023). Androgens and women.Springer Nature. Retrieved October 30, 2024, from https://link.springer.com/chapter/10.1007/978-3-031-31501-5_20

"**Estrogen dominance occurs when there is an excess of estrogen relative to progesterone in the body:**" High Estrogen: Causes, Symptoms, Dominance & Treatment. (n.d.). *Cleveland Clinic*. Retrieved October 30, 2024.

"Low levels of progesterone can result in irregular periods, mood changes, and difficulty conceiving:" Low Progesterone: Causes, Symptoms, Tests & Treatment. (n.d.). *Cleveland Clinic*. Retrieved October 30, 2024.

"**The thyroid gland produces hormones that regulate metabolism, energy levels, and body temperature:**" Hypothyroidism (Underactive Thyroid): Symptoms & Treatment. (n.d.). *Cleveland Clinic*. Retrieved October 30, 2024.

"**Cortisol is a hormone released by the adrenal glands in response to stress:**" Chronic Stress and the HPA Axis: Clinical Assessment and Therapeutic Considerations. (n.d.). *National Center for Biotechnology Information*. Retrieved October 30, 2024.

Cause and Effect Estrogen Dominance: Amy Myers MD. (n.d.). Estrogen dominance: Symptoms, causes & solutions. *Amy Myers MD*. Retrieved October 30, 2024, from https://www.amymyersmd.com/blogs/articles/estrogen-dominance-causes

Cleveland Clinic. (n.d.). High estrogen: Causes, symptoms, dominance & treatment. *Cleveland Clinic*. Retrieved October 30, 2024, from https://my.clevelandclinic.org/health/diseases/22363-high-estrogen

Dr. Will Cole. (n.d.). Causes & treatments for estrogen dominance. *Dr. Will Cole*. Retrieved October 30, 2024, from https://drwillcole.com/hormone-health/estrogen-dominance

Causes and Effects of Progesterone Deficiency: Cleveland Clinic. (n.d.). Low progesterone: Causes, symptoms, tests & treatment. *Cleveland Clinic*. Retrieved October 30, 2024, from https://my.clevelandclinic.org/health/diseases/24613-low-progesterone

Healthline. (n.d.). Low progesterone: Causes, symptoms, and treatment. *Healthline*. Retrieved October 30, 2024, from
https://www.healthline.com/health/womens-health/low-progesterone

Healthgrades. (n.d.). Low progesterone: Definition, symptoms, causes, treatment. *Healthgrades*. Retrieved October 30, 2024, from
https://www.healthgrades.com/right-care/womens-health/low-progesterone

HealthyWomen. (n.d.). Low progesterone symptoms. *HealthyWomen*. Retrieved October 30, 2024, from https://www.healthywomen.org/your-health/low-progesterone.

"Endocrine-disrupting chemicals (EDCs) are substances that can mimic, block, or interfere with the body's natural hormones:" National Institute of Environmental Health Sciences. (n.d.). Endocrine Disruptors. *National Institutes of Health*. Retrieved October 30, 2024, from
https://www.niehs.nih.gov/health/topics/agents/endocrine

"In the 1940s and 1950s, scientists first observed adverse reproductive effects in wildlife exposed to industrial chemicals such as dichlorodiphenyltrichloroethane (DDT) and polychlorinated biphenyls (PCBs).:" International Institute for Sustainable Development. (n.d.). Environmental effects of DDT and PCBs. *IISD Reporting Services*. Retrieved October 30, 2024, from https://enb.iisd.org/journal/wwf.html

"disrupt hormonal balance in humans and even wildlife:" "Multiomics reveal non-alcoholic fatty liver disease in rats following chronic exposure to an ultra-low dose of Roundup herbicide." Mesnage, R., Renney, G., Séralini, G. E., Ward, M., & Antoniou, M. N. (2017). Multiomics reveal non-alcoholic fatty liver disease in rats following chronic exposure to an ultra-low dose of Roundup herbicide. *Scientific Reports*, 7, 39328. https://doi.org/10.1038/srep39328

"Potential toxic effects of glyphosate and its commercial formulations below regulatory limits." Mesnage, R., Defarge, N., Spiroux de Vendômois, J., & Séralini, G.

"Since then, numerous studies have investigated the mechanisms by which EDCs disrupt hormonal balance:" National Institute of

205

Environmental Health Sciences. (n.d.). Endocrine Disruptors. *National Institutes of Health*. Retrieved October 30, 2024, from
https://www.niehs.nih.gov/health/topics/agents/endocrine

"Some studies have indicated that glyphosate can bind to estrogen receptors, potentially disrupting the body's hormone regulation:"
Thongprakaisang, S., Thiantanawat, A., Rangkadilok, N., Suriyo, T., & Satayavivad, J. (2013). Glyphosate induces human breast cancer cells growth via estrogen receptors. Food and Chemical Toxicology, 59, 129-136. https://doi.org/10.1016/j.fct.2013.05.057

Gore, A. C., Chappell, V. A., Fenton, S. E., Flaws, J. A., Nadal, A., Prins, G. S., ... & Zoeller, R. T. (2015). EDC-2: The Endocrine Society's Second Scientific Statement on Endocrine-Disrupting Chemicals. Endocrine Reviews, 36(6), E1-E150. DOI: 10.1210/er.2015-1010

DiGangi, J., Schettler, T., Cobbing, M., & Rossi, M. (2015). Chem Fatale: The Health Impacts of Toxic Chemicals on Women. Women's Voices for the Earth. Available at: https://www.womensvoices.org/wp-content/uploads/2015/10/Chem-Fata-Report.pdf

Bisphenol A (BPA): Mayo Clinic. (n.d.). BPA health risks: What is BPA, and what are the concerns? *Mayo Clinic*. Retrieved October 30, 2024, from
https://www.mayoclinic.org/healthy-lifestyle/nutrition-and-healthy-eating/expert-answers/bpa/faq-20058331

Phthalates: National Institute of Environmental Health Sciences. (n.d.). Phthalates. *National Institutes of Health*. Retrieved October 30, 2024, from https://www.niehs.nih.gov/health/topics/agents/phthalates/index.cfm

Parabens: U.S. Food and Drug Administration. (2023). Parabens in cosmetics. *FDA*. Retrieved October 30, 2024, from
https://www.fda.gov/cosmetics/cosmetic-ingredients/parabens-cosmetics

Fragrances: Breast Cancer Prevention Partners. (2022). Fragrance chemicals and their effects. *Breast Cancer Prevention Partners*. Retrieved October 30, 2024, from https://www.bcpp.org/resource/fragrance-chemicals

Triclosan: U.S. Food and Drug Administration. (2022). Triclosan: What consumers should know. *FDA*. Retrieved October 30, 2024, from https://www.fda.gov/consumers/consumer-updates/triclosan-what-consumers-should-know

Glyphosate: National Pesticide Information Center. (2019). Glyphosate: General fact sheet. *NPIC*. Retrieved October 30, 2024, from http://npic.orst.edu/factsheets/glyphogen.html

"Silicone is a safer alternative to plastics:" Food & Wine. (n.d.). Why you should ditch plastic for silicone. Retrieved October 27, 2024, from https://www.foodandwine.com/lifestyle/kitchen/silicone-baking-mats-vs-plastic

Silicone Kitchenware. (n.d.). Is silicone safe for cooking? Retrieved October 27, 2024, from https://www.silicone-kitchenware.com/blog/is-silicone-safe-for-cooking/

Green Matters. (n.d.). Silicone vs. plastic: Which is better for the environment? Retrieved October 27, 2024, from https://www.greenmatters.com/p/silicone-vs-plastic-environmental-impact

The Spruce Eats. (n.d.). Is silicone safe for cooking? Retrieved October 27, 2024, from https://www.thespruceeats.com/is-silicone-safe-for-cooking-1388541

Chapter 4: Sisterhood, The Red Tent and the Moon

"Menstrual rituals around the world provide insight into cultural practices, beliefs, and traditions related to menstruation:"
The Fornix. (n.d.). 5 menstrual rituals around the world and what they can teach us. *The Fornix Blog*. Retrieved October 30, 2024, from https://blog.flexfits.com/menstrual-rituals-around-the-world/

"In certain Native American cultures, coming-of-age rituals for young women:" The Conversation. (2020, February 7). How a Native American coming of age ritual is making a comeback. *The Conversation*. Retrieved October 30, 2024, from https://theconversation.com/how-a-native-american-coming-of-age-ritual-is-making-a-comeback-130524#

The Red Tent: Diamant, A. (1997). *The Red Tent.* Picador.

"Ancient Hawaiian chants and stories reflect the sacredness of menstrual practices, deeply rooted in mythological traditions and respect for female life cycles." Beckwith, M. W. (1981). *The Kumulipo: A Hawaiian creation chant.* University of Hawaii Press.
Beckwith, M. W. (1970). *Hawaiian mythology.* University of Hawaii Press.

Kalakaua, D. (1990). *The legends and myths of Hawaii: The fables and folklore of a strange people.* Mutual Publishing.

"Menstrual huts or caves, used during menstruation in some cultures, reflect isolation practices based on beliefs around menstruation." PLOS Global Public Health. (2022). Menstrual isolation and public health concerns. *PLOS Global Public Health, 2*(7), e0000355. https://doi.org/10.1371/journal.pgph.0000355

Lancet Regional Health–Americas. (2022). Menstrual health: A neglected public health problem. *The Lancet Regional Health–Americas, 15*, 100399. https://doi.org/10.1016/j.lana.2022.100399

"Period poverty." Jaafar, H., Ismail, S. Y., & Azzeri, A. (2023). Period poverty: A neglected public health issue. *Korean Journal of Family Medicine, 44*(4), 183–188. https://doi.org/10.4082/kjfm.22.0206

"UNICEF highlights the importance of menstrual hygiene products." UNICEF. (n.d.). Menstrual hygiene products. *UNICEF Supply Division.* Retrieved October 30, 2024, from https://www.unicef.org/supply/menstrual-hygiene-products

"Myths around menstruation in India are widespread, often leading to restrictive practices that impact women's well-being and dignity." Narayan, K. A., & Srinivasa, D. K. (2015). Menstruation-related myths in India: Strategies for combating them. *Journal of Family Medicine and Primary Care, 4*(2), 184–186. https://doi.org/10.4103/2249-4863.154627

"The lunar cycle has long been associated with menstrual cycles, influencing traditional beliefs about female rhythms and their connection to nature." Zimecki, M. (2006). The lunar cycle: Effects on human and animal behavior and physiology. *Neuro Endocrinology Letters, 27*(4), 385–392. PMID: 16407788

"Some believe syncing menstrual cycles with the moon—either full or new moon—aligns one's cycle with natural rhythms, fostering a connection with nature." Yoga Goddess. (n.d.). Should your period land on the full moon or the new moon to be in sync with nature? *Yoga Goddess*. Retrieved October 30, 2024, from https://yogagoddess.ca/should-your-period-land-on-the-full-moon-or-the-new-moon-to-be-in-sync-with-nature/

"In mythology, female archetypes associated with the moon and menstrual cycles represent powerful forces in women's lives. Bolen, J. S. (1984). *Goddesses in Everywoman: Thirteen powerful archetypes in women's lives*. Harper & Row.

Chapter 5: Cyclical Rhythms and The Menstrual Cycle

"The story of Demeter and Persephone highlights the cyclical rhythms of nature, paralleling the menstrual cycle and themes of rebirth and transformation."Madeleine. (2019, September 13). Demeter and Persephone from Greek mythology. Theoi Project. Retrieved October 30, 2024, from https://www.theoi.com/articles/what-is-the-demeter-and-persephone-story-summarized/

"The flooding of the Nile River in ancient Egypt was seen as a cycle of renewal, echoing the regenerative processes of the menstrual cycle." Calvert, A. (n.d.). Ancient Egypt, an introduction. Khan Academy. Retrieved October 30, 2024, from https://www.khanacademy.org/humanities/ap-art-history/ancient-mediterranean-ap/ancient-egypt-ap/a/ancient-egypt-an-introduction

"Chinese philosophy, particularly Taoism, emphasizes the balance of Yin and Yang, mirroring the dualistic nature of the menstrual cycle phases." Abbas, S. T. (2024). Harmony in duality: Exploring the philosophical connections between Yin-Yang in Chinese thought and dualism in Western philosophy. Indonesian Journal of Interdisciplinary Research in Science and Technology (MARCOPOLO), 2(2), 159–170. https://doi.org/10.55927/marcopolo.v2i2.7965

"In Hindu cosmology, cycles of creation and destruction are linked to the cosmic order, similar to the reproductive and menstrual cycles." International Journal of Research Publication and Reviews. (2023). The creation of the universe with respect to Hindu methodology and scientific cosmology. International Journal of Research Publication and Reviews, 4(2), 574–583.

"The menstrual cycle consists of four distinct phases, each regulated by complex hormonal changes." Cleveland Clinic. (n.d.). Menstrual cycle. Cleveland Clinic. Retrieved October 30, 2024, from https://my.clevelandclinic.org/health/articles/10132-menstrual-cycle

"Ovulation is tightly regulated by a hormonal feedback loop between the brain and the ovaries." Reed, B. G., & Carr, B. R. (2018). The normal menstrual cycle and the control of ovulation. In Feingold K. R., Anawalt B., Blackman M. R. et al. (Eds.), Endotext. MDText.com, Inc.

"Premenstrual syndrome (PMS) symptoms vary widely and may impact quality of life." Mayo Clinic Staff. (2022). Premenstrual syndrome (PMS). Mayo Clinic. Retrieved October 30, 2024, from https://www.mayoclinic.org/diseases-conditions/premenstrual-syndrome/symptoms-causes/syc-20376780

"Cultural perceptions of menstruation shape attitudes and practices, sometimes contributing to menstrual shame." McHugh, M. (2020). Menstrual shame: Exploring the role of 'menstrual moaning'. In The Palgrave Handbook of Critical Menstruation Studies (Chapter 32). https://doi.org/10.1007/978-981-15-0614-7_32

"Supporting the body through each menstrual phase with diet and lifestyle adjustments may enhance well-being." Vitti, A. (2023, June 16). The menstrual phase: Support your body with The Cycle Syncing Method®. FLO Living. Retrieved October 30, 2024, from https://floliving.com/blog/menstrual-phase

"Menstrual blood loss can lead to iron deficiency, particularly if dietary iron intake is insufficient." Coyne, C. (2018). Menstrual health: Understanding iron deficiency and anemia. Women's Health Journal, 54(3), 215–220.

"Iron is essential for various bodily functions and maintaining adequate levels is crucial, especially for menstruating women." National Institutes of Health. (2020). Iron: Fact sheet for health professionals. Office of Dietary Supplements. Retrieved October 30, 2024, from https://ods.od.nih.gov/factsheets/Iron-HealthProfessional/

"Understanding what's normal in the menstrual cycle can help in identifying potential health concerns." Mayo Clinic. (2016). Menstrual cycle: What's normal, what's not. Mayo Clinic. Retrieved October 30, 2024, from https://www.mayoclinic.org/healthy-lifestyle/womens-health/in-depth/menstrual-cycle/art-20047186

"FSH levels are assessed to evaluate ovarian function and reproductive health." MedlinePlus. (2019). Follicle-stimulating hormone (FSH) levels test. MedlinePlus. Retrieved October 30, 2024, from https://medlineplus.gov/lab-tests/follicle-stimulating-hormone-fsh-levels-test/

"Magnesium plays a role in numerous physiological functions, including hormone regulation." Guerrera, M. P., Volpe, S. L., & Mao, J. J. (2009). Therapeutic uses of magnesium. American Family Physician, 80(2), 157–162.

"Vitamin B6 has been shown to alleviate some symptoms of premenstrual syndrome." Effects of vitamin B6 on premenstrual syndrome: A systematic review and meta-analysis. (2016). Volume, 9(3), 1346–1353.

"Omega-3 fatty acids have anti-inflammatory properties that may support menstrual health." Calder, P. C. (2010). Omega-3 fatty acids and inflammatory processes. Nutrients, 2(3), 355–374. https://doi.org/10.3390/nu2030355

"Intermittent fasting with windows of 14 to 16 hours may impact women's hormones and health." Pelz, M. (n.d.). Women and fasting myths. Dr. Mindy Pelz. Retrieved October 30, 2024, from https://drmindypelz.com/women-and-fasting-myths/

"LH testing can help assess fertility and menstrual health." Swiner, C. N. (2022, September 2). Luteinizing hormone (LH) test. WebMD. Retrieved October 30, 2024.

"Vitamin D is essential for bone health and immune function." National Institutes of Health. (n.d.). Vitamin D: Fact sheet for health professionals. Office of Dietary Supplements. Retrieved October 30, 2024, from https://ods.od.nih.gov/factsheets/VitaminD-HealthProfessional/

"Morning light exposure positively affects circadian rhythms and mood." Sleep Medicine Reviews. (2017). Effects of morning light exposure on circadian rhythms and mood in healthy individuals. Sleep Medicine Reviews, 35, 23–30. https://doi.org/10.1016/j.smrv.2016.07.002

"Morning light exposure helps regulate sleep cycles, supporting a healthy circadian rhythm." Harvard Health Publishing. (n.d.). Morning light exposure: The springboard to a good night's sleep. Harvard Health Publishing. Retrieved October 30, 2024, from https://www.health.harvard.edu/staying-healthy/morning-light-exposure

"Natural red light has been studied for its impact on mood and circadian rhythms." Journal of Sleep Research. (2020). The effects of natural red light on sleep, mood, and circadian rhythms in humans: A systematic review. Journal of Sleep Research, 29(5).

"Carbohydrates are the body's primary energy source, fueling many metabolic processes." Holesh, J. E., Aslam, S., & Martin, A. (2023). Physiology, carbohydrates. In StatPearls. StatPearls Publishing.

"Research indicates that caffeine affects estrogen, cortisol, and insulin levels." National Institutes of Health. (n.d.). Study on caffeine and estrogen levels. HCP Live. Retrieved October 30, 2024, from https://www.nih.gov/news-events/news-releases/nih-study-shows-caffeine-consumption-linked-estrogen-changes
Naturopathic Doctor Phoenix. (n.d.). Research on caffeine's effects on cortisol, insulin, and SHBG. Naturopathic Doctor Phoenix. Retrieved October 30, 2024, from https://www.ncbi.nlm.nih.gov/pmc/articles/PMC3012180/

Chapter 6: Origins of Seed Cycling

"Ancient healing traditions:"Elendu, C. (2024). The evolution of ancient healing practices: From shamanism to Hippocratic medicine: A review. Medicine, 103(28), Article e39005.

"Seeds have long been utilized in Ayurveda for their medicinal properties and are integral to various therapeutic practices." Epstein, D. M. (1997). Ayurvedic medicine: A comprehensive guide. The American Institute of Vedic Studies.

"Seed cycling is a natural practice believed to support hormonal balance through the rotational use of specific seeds during different phases of the menstrual cycle." St. Luke's Health. (n.d.). What is seed cycling, and does it work? Retrieved October 30, 2024, from www.stlukeshealth.org/resources/seed-cycling-and-how-it-works

"Flaxseed, an ancient medicinal food, continues to be valued for its functional health benefits." Kaur, C., & Kapoor, H. C. (2014). Flax and flaxseed oil: An ancient medicine & modern functional food. Journal of Food Science and Technology, 51(9), 1633–1653.

"Sesame seeds are a nutrient-dense food with a long history in traditional medicine and modern nutrition." FoodPrint. (n.d.). Sesame: Real food. FoodPrint. Retrieved October 30, 2024, from https://foodprint.org/real-food/sesame/

"Extra virgin olive oil, rich in healthy fats and antioxidants, is widely"Healthline. (2023, September 18). Extra virgin olive oil: Nutrition, benefits, and cooking tips. Healthline. Retrieved October 30, 2024.

"Sunflower oil has been a part of human nutrition since ancient times, evolving with dietary practices."Tsimidou, M. Z., & Lazos, E. S. (2020). Sunflower oil: From ancient times to modern days. OCL - Oilseeds and fats, Crops and Lipids, 27(1), 15. https://doi.org/10.1051/ocl/2020028

"Pumpkin seeds are nutrient-rich and have various health benefits." King, L. M. (2024, January 4). Pumpkin seeds: How healthy are they? Healthline. Retrieved October 30, 2024.

"Experts caution against the consumption of highly processed sunflower oil due to its potential health risks." Hyman, M. (2020). Food: What the heck should I cook? Little, Brown Spark.
Weil, A. (2019). The true food cookbook: 125 recipes for optimal wellness. HarperOne. Perlmutter, D. (2016). Brain maker: The power of gut microbes to heal and protect your brain for life. Little, Brown and Company.
Shanahan, C. (2017). Deep nutrition: Why your genes need traditional food. Flatiron Books.

"Pumpkin seed oil has shown potential benefits for managing urinary disorders." Nishimura, M., Ohkawara, T., Sato, H., Takeda, H., & Nishihira, J. (2014). Pumpkin seed oil extracted from Cucurbita maxima improves urinary disorder in human overactive bladder. Journal of Traditional and Complementary Medicine, 4(1), 72–74. https://doi.org/10.4103/2225-4110.124355

"Sesame ingestion can influence sex hormones and has antioxidant properties." Wu, W. H., Kang, Y. P., Wang, N. H., Jou, H. J., & Wang, T. A. (2006). Sesame ingestion affects sex hormones, antioxidant status, and blood lipids in postmenopausal women. The Journal of Nutrition, 136(5), 1270–1275. https://doi.org/10.1093/jn/136.5.1270

"Flax and flaxseed oil have ancient medicinal uses and continue to serve as modern functional foods." Goyal, A., Sharma, V., Upadhyay, N., Gill, S., & Sihag, M. (2014). Flax and flaxseed oil: An ancient medicine & modern functional food. Journal of Food Science and Technology, 51(9), 1633–1653.

"Seed cycling is a holistic approach aimed at supporting hormone balance by synchronizing seed intake with the menstrual cycle phases." Brighten, J. (2019, January 9). Seed cycling: A natural approach to hormone balance. Dr. Brighten. Retrieved October 30, 2024, from https://drbrighten.com/seed-cycling

"Using the Cycle Syncing Method® helps align diet and lifestyle with hormonal phases to enhance well-being." Vitti, A. (2020). In the flow: Unlock your hormonal advantage and revolutionize your life. Hay House.

"Seed cycling may support hormonal balance, particularly for women experiencing menstrual irregularities." The Natural Nutritionist. (2023, March). Seed cycling: A guide to balancing hormones. The Natural Nutritionist. Retrieved October 30, 2024, from https://thenaturalnutritionist.com/seed-cycling

"Seed cycling offers a structured approach to managing hormone balance through diet." Hyman, M. (2022, June 20). Seed cycling 101: The ultimate guide to balancing hormones. Dr. Hyman. Retrieved October 30, 2024, from https://drhyman.com/blog/2022/06/20/seed-cycling-101-the-ultimate-guide-to-balancing-hormones/

Chapter 7: Seed Cycling Nutrients, Science and Research

"For many years, women were often excluded from clinical trials, leading to gaps in understanding women's health and treatment outcomes." National Institutes of Health. (1994). Guidelines on the inclusion of women and minorities as subjects in clinical research. National Institutes of Health. Retrieved October 30, 2024, from https://grants.nih.gov/grants/guide/notice-files/not94-100.html

"Biases in biomedical research have historically led to underrepresentation of female biology in neuroscience studies." Beery, A., & Zucker, I. (2011). Sex bias in neuroscience and biomedical research. Neuroscience & Biobehavioral Reviews, 35(3), 565–572.

"The historical exclusion of women from clinical trials has had lasting implications for women's health." Eisenberg, D. (2018). The historical exclusion of women from clinical trials: The implications for women's health. Women's Health Issues, 28(4), 259–262.

"In recent years, the NIH has implemented guidelines to include sex and gender:" Meyer, K., & Nussbaum, M. (2016). The role of sex and gender in health research: The NIH's approach to inclusion. Journal of Women's Health, 25(8), 716–720.

"Women's health research has evolved significantly, though historically it was often neglected." Rosenberg, L., & Freedman, L. S. (2018). The history of women's health research. American Journal of Public Health, 108(2), 191–194.

"Seed cycling, rooted in Chinese medicine, is believed to support hormone balance and fertility." Bentolila, S. (2021, July 21). Seed cycling or fertility: Chinese medicine's perspective. Acupuncture Taproot. Retrieved October 30, 2024, from https://www.acupuncturetaproot.com/post/seed-cycling-for-fertility-chinese-medicine-s-perspective

"Combined seeds like pumpkin, sunflower, sesame, and flaxseed may reduce inflammation and support menstrual health in PCOS." Rasheed, N., Ahmed, A., Nosheen, F., Imran, A., Islam, F., Noreen, R., Chauhan, A., Shah, M. A., & Ali, Y. A. (2023). Effectiveness of combined seeds as adjunct therapy to treat polycystic ovary syndrome in females. Food Science & Nutrition, 11(6), 3385–3393.

"Flaxseed's anti-estrogen effects vary, with recent studies questioning the consistency of this effect." Kajla, P., Sharma, A., & Sood, D. R. (2015). Flaxseed—a potential functional food source. Journal of Food Science and Technology, 52(4), 1857–1871. https://doi.org/10.1007/s13197-014-1293-y

"Flaxseed meal is often derived from byproducts, differing nutritionally from whole flaxseed." Manitoba Flax Milling Co. (n.d.). Flaxseed meal vs. milled flaxseed: There's a difference. Manitoba Flax. Retrieved October 30, 2024.

"Flaxseed has varying effects on estrogen targets, as observed in pre-neoplastic studies." Dikshit, A., Gao, C., Small, C., Hales, K., & Hales, D. B. (2016). Flaxseed and its components differentially affect estrogen targets in pre-neoplastic hen ovaries. Journal of Steroid Biochemistry and Molecular Biology, 159, 73–85. https://doi.org/10.1016/j.jsbmb.2016.02.028

"Flaxseed may have positive effects on glycemic control in individuals with prediabetes and type 2 diabetes." Villarreal-Renteria, A. I., Herrera-Echauri, D. D., Rodríguez-Rocha, N. P., Zuñiga, L. Y., Muñoz-Valle, J. F., García-Arellano, S., & Macedo-Ojeda, G. (2022). Effect of flaxseed supplementation on glycemic control and insulin resistance in prediabetes and type 2 diabetes: A systematic review and meta-analysis of randomized controlled trials. Complementary Therapies in Medicine, 70, 102852. https://doi.org/10.1016/j.ctim.2022.102852

"**Flaxseed ingestion may impact the menstrual cycle, influencing cycle length and symptoms.**" Phipps, W. R., Martini, M. C., Lampe, J. W., Slavin, J. L., & Kurzer, M. S. (1993). Effect of flax seed ingestion on the menstrual cycle. Journal of Clinical Endocrinology & Metabolism, 77(5), 1215–1219. https://doi.org/10.1210/jcem.77.5.8077314

"**Dietary phytoestrogens, including those in flaxseed, may influence hormonal health.**" Rietjens, I. M. C. M., Louisse, J., & Beekmann, K. (2016). The potential health effects of dietary phytoestrogens. British Journal of Pharmacology, 174(11), 1263–1280. https://doi.org/10.1111/bph.13622

"**The corpus luteum plays a crucial role in supporting early pregnancy by producing progesterone.**" Smith. (2017). Corpus luteum: Function, formation, and cysts. Medical News Today. Retrieved October 30, 2024, from https://www.medicalnewstoday.com/articles/320433

"**The lignans in flaxseeds have been associated with longer luteal phases in some studies.**" Desmawati, D., & Sulastri, D. (2019). Phytoestrogens and their health effect. Open Access Macedonian Journal of Medical Sciences, 7(3), 495–499. https://doi.org/10.3889/oamjms.2019.086

"**Lignans may help balance sex hormones and reduce inflammation.**" Musazadeh, V., Nazari, A., Natami, M., Hajhashemy, Z., Kazemi, K. S., Torabi, F., Moridpour, A. H., Vajdi, M., & Askari, G. (2023). The effect of flaxseed supplementation on sex hormone profile in adults: A systematic review and meta-analysis. Frontiers in Nutrition, 10, Article 1222584. https://doi.org/10.3389/fnut.2023.1222584

"**High lignan intake has been linked to a lower risk of postmenopausal breast cancer.**" Zaineddin, A. K., Buck, K., Vrieling, A., Heinz, J., Flesch-Janys, D., Linseisen, J., & Chang-Claude, J. (2012). The association between dietary lignans, phytoestrogen-rich foods, and fiber intake and postmenopausal breast cancer risk: A German case-control study. Nutrition and Cancer, 64(5), 652–665. https://doi.org/10.1080/01635581.2012.683227

"PCOS has long-term health consequences, including metabolic and reproductive issues." Daniilidis, A., & Dinas, K. (2009). Long-term health consequences of polycystic ovarian syndrome: A review analysis. Hippokratia, 13(2), 90–92.

"Nutraceutical interventions, like seed cycling, show promise in managing PCOS symptoms." Aslam, M., Shauket, R., Yousaf, Z., & Tehzeeb, K. (2021). Nutraceutical intervention of seeds in the treatment of polycystic ovarian syndrome; A systematic review. Pakistan BioMedical Journal, 4(2). https://doi.org/10.54393/pbmj.v4i2.100

Chapter 8: Seed Cycling Benefits and How to Get Started

"A regular menstrual cycle typically lasts between 21 to 35 days, with ovulation occurring midway." Mayo Clinic. (n.d.). Menstrual cycle: What's normal, what's not. *Mayo Clinic*. Retrieved October 30, 2024, from https://www.mayoclinic.org/healthy-lifestyle/womens-health/in-depth/menstrual-cycle/art-20047186

"Seed cycling involves the use of specific seeds to support hormonal balance and improve menstrual health." Hall, A. (2017). Seed cycling for hormonal balance. *Herbal Academy*. Retrieved October 30, 2024, from https://theherbalacademy.com/seed-cycling-for-hormonal-balance/

"Seed cycling for hormone balance helps support natural hormone production and is safe for anyone to use." Neuzil, A. (2017). Seed cycling for hormone balance. *To Health With That*. Retrieved October 30, 2024.

"Seed cycling, an approach to balancing hormones through diet, has gained popularity for its perceived benefits." Jardim, N. (n.d.). Seed cycling. *The Period Girl*. Retrieved October 30, 2024, from https://nicolejardim.com/seed-cycling/

"The practice of seed cycling is said to align with different phases of the menstrual cycle to support hormonal health." Natural Fertility Info. (n.d.). Seed cycling for menstrual cycle. *Natural Fertility Info*. Retrieved

October 30, 2024, from https://natural-fertility-info.com/seed-cycling-for-menstrual-cycle.html

"Seed cycling is promoted for women with irregular or absent periods as a method to support hormonal regulation." No Period Now. (n.d.). Seed cycling for no period. *No Period Now*. Retrieved October 30, 2024, from https://www.noperiodnowwhat.com/research/seed-cycling-for-no-period-nope

"This guide on seed cycling offers insights into balancing hormones naturally through dietary seeds." The Chalkboard. (n.d.). How to seed cycle for your period & hormone health. *The Chalkboard Magazine*. Retrieved October 30, 2024.

"Seed cycling may be beneficial for menopausal hormones, supporting a smoother transition." Brighton, J. (n.d.). Seed cycling for menopausal hormones. *Dr. Jolene Brighton*. Retrieved October 30, 2024, from https://drbrighten.com/seed-cycling-menopausal-hormones/

"Omega-3 fatty acids play a role in skin health, supporting moisture retention and reducing inflammation." Burr, G. O., & Burr, M. M. (1930). On the nature and role of the fatty acids essential in nutrition. *Journal of Biological Chemistry, 86*, 587–621.

"Essential fatty acids are important for maintaining healthy skin and supporting overall skin function." Linus Pauling Institute. (n.d.). Essential fatty acids and skin health. *Linus Pauling Institute*. Retrieved October 30, 2024, from https://lpi.oregonstate.edu/mic/health-disease/skin-health/essential-fatty-acids

"Seed cycling is often used to alleviate PMS symptoms like breast tenderness and mood swings." Hormones and Balance. (n.d.). How to use seed rotation to rebalance your menstrual cycle. *Hormones and Balance*. Retrieved October 30, 2024, from https://hormonesbalance.com/articles/how-to-use-seed-rotation-to-rebalance-your-menstrual-cycle/

"Dietary flaxseed and omega-3 supplements have been shown to help reduce cyclical breast tenderness in women."

Vaziri, F., Zamani Lari, M., Samsami Dehaghani, A., Salehi, M., Sadeghpour, H., Akbarzadeh, M., & Zare, N. (2014). Comparing the effects of dietary flaxseed and omega-3 fatty acids supplement on cyclical mastalgia in Iranian women: A randomized clinical trial. *International Journal of Family Medicine*, Article 174532. https://doi.org/10.1155/2014/174532

"Seed cycling may support weight management as part of a balanced hormonal approach." Phipps, W. R., Martini, M. C., Lampe, J. W., Slavin, J. L., & Kurzer, M. S. (1993). Effect of flax seed ingestion on the menstrual cycle. *Journal of Clinical Endocrinology and Metabolism, 77*(5), 1215–1219. https://doi.org/10.1210/jcem.77.5.8077314

"Omega-3 fatty acids are recognized for their potential health benefits, including supporting hormone health." Kajla, P., Sharma, A., & Sood, D. R. (2015). Flaxseed—a potential functional food source. *Journal of Food Science and Technology, 52*(4), 1857–1871. https://doi.org/10.1007/s13197-014-1293-y

"In Chinese herbology, seeds are traditionally used to support fertility and hormonal balance." Acupuncture Taproot. (n.d.). Seed cycling for fertility: A Chinese medicine perspective. *Acupuncture Taproot*. Retrieved October 30, 2024.

"Phytoestrogens found in seeds may contribute to hormone health by interacting with estrogen receptors." Desmawati, D., & Sulastri, D. (2019). Phytoestrogens and their health effect. *Open Access Macedonian Journal of Medical Sciences, 7*(3), 495–499. https://doi.org/10.3889/oamjms.2019.086

"The moon's phases are believed to have an influence on hormonal cycles and rhythms in the body." ScienceDirect. (n.d.). Lunar cycle. *ScienceDirect*. Retrieved October 30, 2024, from https://www.sciencedirect.com/topics/medicine-and-dentistry/lunar-cycle

"Phytic acid, found in some seeds, can impact mineral absorption but also has potential health benefits." Kumar, V., Sinha, A. K., Makkar, H. P., & Becker, K. (2010). Dietary roles of phytate and phytase in human

nutrition. *Food Chemistry, 120*(4), 945–959.
https://doi.org/10.1016/j.foodchem.2009.11.052

"Cold milling is a technique that helps preserve the nutritional value of seeds by preventing heat damage." Thompson, L. U. (1993). Potential health benefits and problems associated with antinutrients in foods. *Food Research International, 26*(2), 131–149.

"Ovulation can be tracked through various symptoms:" Fields, L. (2024, June 2). Ovulation symptoms. *WebMD*. Medically reviewed by Poonam Sachdev. Retrieved October 30, 2024, from https://www.webmd.com/baby/am-i-ovulating

Chapter 9: Seed Cycling for PMS and Teens

"Premenstrual syndrome (PMS) includes a variety of symptoms that affect women before their menstrual periods." Mayo Clinic Staff. (2022). Premenstrual syndrome (PMS). Mayo Clinic. Retrieved October 30, 2024, from https://www.mayoclinic.org/diseases-conditions/premenstrual-syndrome/symptoms-causes/syc-20376780

"Supporting the body's hormonal transition off birth control can help minimize side effects." Brighten, J. (2019). Beyond the Pill: A 30-Day Program to Balance Your Hormones, Reclaim Your Body, and Reverse the Dangerous Side Effects of the Birth Control Pill. HarperOne.

"PMS and period-related issues are prevalent worldwide, impacting many women's health and quality of life." Gao, M., Zhang, H., Gao, G., Cheng, X., Sun, Y., Qiao, M., & Gao, D. (2022). Global and regional prevalence and burden for premenstrual syndrome and premenstrual dysphoric disorder. Medicine (Baltimore), 101(1).

"Mood changes are often experienced during different phases of the menstrual cycle." Jennis. (2021). How does your mood change across your menstrual cycle? Jennis.com. Retrieved October 30, 2024, from https://www.jennis.com/blog/cyclemapping/how-does-your-mood-change-across-your-menstrual-cycle/

"Cultural stigma around menstruation can lead to menstrual shame, affecting women's mental health." McHugh, M. (2020). Menstrual shame: Exploring the role of 'menstrual moaning'. In The Palgrave Handbook of Critical Menstruation Studies (Chapter 32). https://doi.org/10.1007/978-981-15-0614-7_32

"PMDD is a severe form of PMS, causing emotional and physical symptoms that disrupt daily life."Mayo Clinic Staff. (2023). Premenstrual dysphoric disorder (PMDD). Mayo Clinic. Retrieved October 30, 2024, from https://www.mayoclinic.org/diseases-conditions/premenstrual-dysphoric-disorder/symptoms-causes/syc-20376780

"Many women report dissatisfaction with how healthcare providers address PMS symptoms."
The Journal of Women's Health. (2018). Premenstrual syndrome and healthcare provider interaction: A study of women's experiences. Journal of Women's Health, 27(5), 630–638. https://doi.org/10.1089/jwh.2017.6671

"Various factors, including hormonal changes, contribute to PMS symptoms."The Cochrane Database of Systematic Reviews. (2019). Hormonal treatments for premenstrual syndrome. Cochrane Database of Systematic Reviews, 2019(2), CD004630. https://doi.org/10.1002/14651858.CD004630.pub5

"Societal attitudes and medical dismissal may influence how women's PMS symptoms are perceived and treated." Psychology of Women Quarterly. (2020). Societal attitudes and medical dismissal of premenstrual symptoms: An analysis. Psychology of Women Quarterly, 44(3), 350–363. https://doi.org/10.1177/0361684320904397

"New advancements in diagnosing and treating PMDD are emerging to improve women's quality of life." The American Journal of Obstetrics and Gynecology. (2021). Advances in the diagnosis and treatment of premenstrual dysphoric disorder. American Journal of Obstetrics and Gynecology, 224(3), 302–310.

"Seed cycling has gained attention as a natural approach to reducing PMS symptoms." Seed Cycle. (n.d.). Seed cycling: A natural approach to

hormone balance. The Seed Cycle™. Retrieved October 30, 2024, from
https://www.theseedcycle.com.au

"Nutritional interventions, including certain micronutrients, may help in managing PMS symptoms." Gordon, M., & Walker, S. (2021). The role of nutritional interventions in managing premenstrual syndrome: A review. Nutrients, 13(3), 929. https://doi.org/10.3390/nu13030929

"Estrogen dominance can play a role in PMS symptoms and other hormone-related conditions." Prior, J. C. (2006). Progesterone for symptomatic perimenopause treatment: A review. Women's Health, 2(1), 17–33.

"Progesterone interacts with GABA receptors, potentially influencing mood and reproductive mood disorders." Smith, S. S., & Woolley, C. S. (2004). GABA and the neurosteroid regulation of reproductive mood disorders. Neuropsychopharmacology, 29, 497–507.

"Oxidative stress and inflammation are influential factors in ovulation and reproductive health." Ruder, E. H., Hartman, T. J., & Goldman, M. B. (2009). Impact of oxidative stress on female fertility. Current Opinion in Obstetrics & Gynecology, 21(3), 219–222. https://doi.org/10.1097/GCO.0b013e32832924ba

"Certain whole foods have anti-inflammatory properties that may alleviate PMS symptoms." Harris, M., & Smith, M. (2018). Dietary patterns and inflammation: Evidence for the anti-inflammatory effects of whole foods. Nutrients, 10(9), 1393. https://doi.org/10.3390/nu10091393

"Liver detoxification processes are involved in estrogen metabolism and may impact inflammation." Lundh, T., Pettersson, H., & Dahlberg, E. (1990). Detoxification of estrogen in the liver: Studies in women with normal and abnormal menstrual cycles. Journal of Steroid Biochemistry, 35(4), 441–446. https://doi.org/10.1016/0022-4731(90)90260-Q

"Deficiencies in magnesium, calcium, and vitamin D have been linked to PMS symptoms." Thys-Jacobs, S. (2000). Micronutrients and the premenstrual syndrome: The case for calcium. Journal of the American

College of Nutrition, 19(2), 220–227.
https://doi.org/10.1080/07315724.2000.10718927

"Stress and cortisol imbalances may worsen PMS symptoms in some women." Hantsoo, L., & Epperson, C. N. (2015). Premenstrual dysphoric disorder: Epidemiology and treatment. Current Psychiatry Reports, 17(11), 87. https://doi.org/10.1007/s11920-015-0638-x

"The gut microbiome plays a significant role in estrogen metabolism, influencing PMS and hormone balance." Plottel, C. S., & Blaser, M. J. (2011). Microbiome and its role in estrogen metabolism. Science, 334(6052), 587–592. https://doi.org/10.1126/science.1208173

"Managing stress through mindfulness may help alleviate some PMS symptoms." Creswell, J. D., & Lindsay, E. K. (2019). Mindfulness and stress management in premenstrual syndrome: An overview. Psychosomatic Medicine, 81(5), 417–425.

"Exposure to environmental toxins, particularly endocrine-disrupting chemicals, may exacerbate PMS symptoms." Rudel, R. A., & Sergeyev, O. (2021). Endocrine-disrupting chemicals in personal care products and their impact on menstrual health. Environmental Health Perspectives, 129(6), 067001.

"Avoiding EDCs in personal care products may benefit hormonal balance and reduce PMS severity." Konieczna, A., Rutkowska, A., & Rachoń, D. (2015). Health risk of exposure to Bisphenol A (BPA). Rocz Panstw Zakl Hig, 66(1), 5–11.

"Hormonal imbalances due to EDC exposure are linked to menstrual issues and PMS." Zota, A. R., Calafat, A. M., & Woodruff, T. J. (2014). Temporal trends in phthalate exposures: Findings from the National Health and Nutrition Examination Survey, 2001–2010. Environmental Health Perspectives, 122(3), 235–241. https://doi.org/10.1289/ehp.1306681

"Certain skincare products contain EDCs that may disrupt hormone function." Dodson, R. E., Nishioka, M., Standley, L. J., Perovich, L. J., Brody, J. G., & Rudel, R. A. (2012). Endocrine disruptors and asthma-associated chemicals in consumer products. Environmental Health Perspectives, 120(7), 935–943.

Chapter 10: Menopause and Seed Cycling

"Throughout history and in various cultures, menopause." Harlow, S. D., & Matanoski, G. M. (1998). The menopause transition: A historical perspective. In *Menopause and the Menopause Transition*. Cambridge University Press.

"Cultural perceptions of menopause vary widely, influencing how women experience and interpret this stage of life." Bowers, B. J., & Thomeer, M. B. (2014). Cultural variations in the experience and perception of menopause: A review of the literature. *Journal of Women's Health, 23*(4), 334–340.

"The menopause experience is shaped by cultural, social, and psychological factors, creating a diverse range of menopausal experiences globally." Miller, J. K., & Marcellin, E. (2020). Menopause in cross-cultural perspective: From ancient wisdom to contemporary practices. *Journal of Cross-Cultural Psychology, 51*(8), 637–652.

"Menopause is often interpreted through a cultural and social lens, with some societies viewing it as a time of increased wisdom and status." Gordon, R., & Lynch, M. (2017). Menopause as a cultural and social construct: Insights from traditional societies. *Anthropology & Medicine, 24*(1), 10–25.

"The meanings of menopause have evolved over time": Gordon, D. H. (2008). The changing meanings of menopause: Historical and cross-cultural perspectives. *Women & Health, 47*(3), 143–162.

"In ancient Greek texts, there is evidence of changing roles for women post-childbearing." Homer. (8th Century BCE). *Homeric Hymns*. Translated by Evelyn-White, Hugh G. Harvard University Press.

"Ancient Greek religious beliefs acknowledged life transitions." Parker, R. (2005). *On Greek Religion*. Cornell University Press.

"In many Indigenous cultures, menopausal women are honoured as wise figures." Eller, C. J. (2007). Cultural and social perspectives on menopause: A comparative study. *Anthropological Journal of European Cultures, 16*(2), 51–69.

"Flaxseed has shown potential in alleviating menopausal symptoms, making it a natural aid for managing menopause." Journal of Women's Health. (2021). The effects of flaxseed on menopausal symptoms: A systematic review. *Journal of Women's Health, 30*(7), 1083–1090.

"The grandmother hypothesis suggests that menopause may have evolved." Stewart, D., & Johnson, L. (2019). The grandmother hypothesis: Evolutionary insights into menopause and grandparenting. *Evolutionary Anthropology, 28*(3), 113–123.

"Clinical insights into perimenopause and menopause highlight the importance of individualized management for symptom relief." Henderson, V. W., & St. John, J. (2018). Perimenopause and menopause: Clinical insights and management. *Menopause, 25*(6), 655–662.

"Flaxseed has been recognized for its health benefits, including potential relief of menopausal symptoms." Miller, P. E., & Nettleton, J. A. (2016). Flaxseed and its health benefits: A systematic review. *Nutrients, 8*(9), 584.

Chapter 11: Seed Cycling for PCOS and Other Conditions

"Polycystic ovary syndrome (PCOS) affects millions of women worldwide" World Health Organization. (2023). Polycystic ovary syndrome. *World Health Organization*. Retrieved October 30, 2024, from https://www.who.int/news-room/fact-sheets/detail/polycystic-ovary-syndrome

"PCOS can lead to long-term health consequences, including increased risk for metabolic and cardiovascular diseases." Daniilidis, A., & Dinas, K. (2009). Long-term health consequences of polycystic ovarian syndrome: A review analysis. *Hippokratia, 13*(2), 90–92.

"The cause of PCOS is not fully understood, but experts suggest a complex interaction of genetic, hormonal, and metabolic factors." Mayo Clinic. (2023). Polycystic ovary syndrome (PCOS). *Mayo Clinic*. Retrieved October 30, 2024.

"Genetic predisposition, hormonal imbalances, and metabolic disruptions are among the primary factors linked to PCOS." Azziz, R., Carmina, E., Dewailly, D., Oppenheimer, G., & Tarlatzis, B. C. (2009). Polycystic ovary syndrome. *Nature Reviews Disease Primers, 1*, 15028.

"Insulin resistance and inflammation are closely associated with PCOS, potentially exacerbating symptoms." Clemente, M., Palomba, S., & Orio, F. (2018). Insulin resistance and PCOS: The role of inflammation. *Journal of Endocrinological Investigation, 41*(8), 885–895.

"Seed cycling has shown promise as a natural intervention for managing PCOS symptoms, according to recent reviews." Aslam, M., Shauket, R., Yousaf, Z., & Tehzeeb, K. (2021). Nutraceutical intervention of seeds in the treatment of polycystic ovarian syndrome; A systematic review. *Pakistan BioMedical Journal, 4*(2). https://doi.org/10.54393/pbmj.v4i2.100

"A 2023 study examined the effects of seed cycling on PCOS and found improvements in hormonal balance and symptom management." Chaudhary, N., & Chiu, T. (2023). The effect of seed cycling on polycystic ovary syndrome: A pilot study. *Nutrients, 15*(14), 3251.

"Nutraceutical elements present in seeds, such as lignans and omega-3 fatty acids, may support hormonal balance in PCOS." Shahnazari, Z., Bagheri, M., & Zadeh, S. S. (2022). Flaxseed and its effects on polycystic ovary syndrome: A review. *Journal of Nutrition and Metabolism, 2022*, 8835454.

"Regular flaxseed ingestion over three months has shown potential in alleviating PCOS symptoms." Therapeutic potential of flaxseed in the treatment of polycystic ovarian syndrome: A review. *International Journal of Pharmaceutical Sciences Review and Research, 31*(1), 140–144.

"Studies indicate that flaxseed supplementation can reduce markers of inflammation and improve endothelial function." Effects of flaxseed supplementation on markers of inflammation and endothelial function: A systematic review and meta-analysis of randomized controlled trials. *Nutrition Journal, 19*(1), 1–15.

"Phytoestrogens in flaxseed may bind to estrogen receptors, helping to balance hormonal levels in women with PCOS." Nutraceutical intervention of seeds in the treatment of polycystic ovarian syndrome: A systematic review. *Pakistan BioMedical Journal, 4*(2), 84–90.

"Omega-3 fatty acids found in seeds, such as flaxseed, offer numerous health benefits including support for cardiovascular health." Miller, P. E., & Nettleton, J. A. (2016). Flaxseed and its health benefits: A systematic review. *Nutrients, 8*(9), 584.

"Flaxseed consumption may aid in lowering cholesterol levels and supporting weight loss efforts." Cruz, A. G., & Amaral, L. A. (2018). Effect of flaxseed consumption on body weight and blood lipid levels in overweight and obese individuals: A meta-analysis. *European Journal of Clinical Nutrition, 72*(9), 1314–1322.

"Flaxseed may have protective effects against certain types of breast cancer, according to recent studies." Zhao, M., & Hu, X. (2020). Protective effects of flaxseed and its components against cancer: A review of recent evidence. *Frontiers in Oncology, 10*, 317.

"Omega-3 fatty acids are beneficial in managing inflammatory conditions, which can include adenomyosis." Liu, Y., & Sun, X. (2020). The role of omega-3 fatty acids in inflammatory conditions: A review. *Frontiers in Nutrition, 7*, 89.

"Omega-3s have been studied for their potential anti-inflammatory effects on endometrial health." Harris, W. S., & Del Gobbo, L. C. (2021). Omega-3 fatty acids and inflammation: Effects on endometrial health. *Nutrition Reviews, 79*(3), 211–228.

"Fibroids, which are benign uterine tumors, can have a range of symptoms and affect many women." Laughlin-Tommaso, S. K., &

Stewart, E. A. (2019). Uterine fibroids: Diagnosis and treatment. *BMJ, 365*, l1777.

"Certain dietary and lifestyle factors may influence fibroid growth, offering a potential approach to management." Cheng, M., & Liu, J. (2020). Diet and lifestyle factors in uterine fibroids: A review. *International Journal of Women's Health, 12*, 1153–1164.

"Research suggests that high dietary fiber intake may reduce the risk of fibroids." Baird, D. D., & Dunson, D. B. (2019). The effect of dietary fiber on fibroid risk: Evidence from epidemiological studies. *American Journal of Epidemiology, 188*(9), 1680–1686. https://doi.org/10.1093/aje/kwz157

"An anti-inflammatory diet may support uterine health and potentially influence fibroid development." Gupta, S., & Nair, V. (2018). Impact of anti-inflammatory diet on uterine health and fibroids. *Journal of Nutritional Science, 7*, e12.

"Selenium plays a crucial role in thyroid health, supporting hormone regulation and thyroid function." Harris, S. S., & Horne, W. C. (2021). The role of selenium in thyroid function: A review of the evidence. *Current Opinion in Endocrinology, Diabetes and Obesity, 28*(4), 345–351.

"Zinc is essential for thyroid health and supports overall endocrine balance." Muller, M., & Hwang, C. H. (2022). Zinc and thyroid health: Implications for clinical practice. *Journal of Clinical Endocrinology & Metabolism, 107*(3), 692–701.

"Nutritional approaches can be valuable in managing thyroid disorders and improving overall thyroid health." Gartner, R., & Papageorgiou, A. (2019). Nutritional approaches to managing thyroid disorders: An overview. *Frontiers in Endocrinology, 10*, 247.

Chapter 12: Seed Cycling Recipes

"Cooking can transform our relationship with food, helping us to engage more mindfully and develop a healthier approach to eating." Arch, J. J., & Landy, L. N. (2019). Mindful emotional eating: Harnessing the psychology of mindfulness for healthy eating. *Frontiers in Psychology, 10*, 2238.

"Cooking has influenced human health and evolutionary pathwaysL., & Liu, J. (2014). The impact of cooking on human health: Evolutionary insights. *Evolutionary Anthropology, 23*(3), 117–129.

"Creative activities, including cooking, positively impact well-being and mental health." *Frontiers in Psychology*. (2018). Creative activities and their impact on well-being: A longitudinal study of cooking and mental health. *Frontiers in Psychology, 9*, Article 2738. https://doi.org/10.3389/fpsyg.2018.02738

"Simple, mindful cooking can be revolutionary, turning food preparation into a joyful, healthful practice." Waters, A. (2007). *The Art of Simple Food: Notes, Lessons, and Recipes from a Delicious Revolution*. Clarkson Potter.

"Rituals during mealtime can enhance the consumption experience, making food more enjoyable." *The Journal of Positive Psychology*. (2013). Rituals enhance the consumption experience: Psychological research on the benefits of rituals during mealtime. *The Journal of Positive Psychology, 8*(6), 461–470. https://doi.org/10.1080/17439760.2013.830760

"Choosing what to cook is crucial for health, encouraging the use of whole, nutrient-dense foods." Hyman, M. (2019). *Food: What the Heck Should I Cook?*. Little, Brown Spark.

"Social eating behaviors can influence weight, with implications for long-term health." Robinson, E., Tobias, T., Shaw, L., Freeman, E., & Higgs, S. (2016). Social eating and weight gain: A prospective study in UK adults. *Appetite, 106*, 261–268. https://doi.org/10.1016/j.appet.2016.07.039

"Rapadura sugar retains more nutrients than refined sugars, making it a nutritious alternative." Reddy, R. P., & Misra, S. S. (2016). Nutritional composition and health benefits of rapadura sugar: An overview. *Journal of Food Science and Technology, 53*(4), 1854–1860.

"Rapadura sugar contains beneficial minerals and antioxidants, adding nutritional value to its sweet flavor." Gonzalez, J. A., & Hernandez, C. J. (2018). Mineral content and antioxidant properties of rapadura sugar. *Food Chemistry, 260*, 174–179.

"Caloric value of food varies by nutrient density, and calorie counting alone can mislead health outcomes." Weaver, L. (2018). *The Calorie Fallacy: How the Calorie Myth Is Ruining Your Life*. Hay House.

"The USDA pioneered calorie measurement, but nutritional quality involves more than calories alone." Atwater, W. O., & Bryant, A. P. (1902). The chemical composition and calorific value of the foods of the United States. *United States Department of Agriculture Bulletin*, 108.

"Determining the best diet for health requires assessing nutrient quality, not just caloric content." Katz, D. L., & Meller, S. (2014). Can we say what diet is best for health? *Annual Review of Public Health, 35*, 83–103.

"Nutrient density should be a focus for health, as it supports both physical and mental well-being." Sweeney, J., & Bernstein, S. (2020). Beyond calories: The role of nutrient density in promoting health. *Journal of Nutrition and Metabolism, 2020*, 752–762.

"Therapeutic dosage guidelines for seeds can maximize their nutritional benefits, including hormonal support." Hodge, A., & Ma, D. (2020). Nutritional benefits of seeds: An overview of therapeutic dosage and efficacy. *Journal of Nutritional Science, 9*, e27.

Index

acne, 32, 82, 87, 100, 106, 108, 117, 120, 128, 142, 143, 144, 146, 147, 148, 149, 162, 165, 167

Adenomyosis, 167

adrenal, 36, 39, 40, 41, 42, 44

alpha-linolenic acid, 95

antioxidants, 16, 26, 92, 103, 167, 175, 176, 196, 205

anxiety, 8, 26, 27, 39, 44, 100, 142, 156, 158

Ayurvedic, 14, 37, 79, 80, 125

blood sugar, 36, 103, 110, 112, 166, 193

bone health, 38, 39, 71, 92

breastfeeding, 41, 128, 134

calcium, 65, 99, 100, 101, 102, 104, 129, 132, 139, 171

Chinese medicine, 14, 125

cholesterol, 38, 92, 103, 110, 111, 166

coffee, 72, 154

cognitive function, 80, 103

collagen, 117, 189

Constipation, 137

cyclical, 53, 56, 61, 62, 70, 74, 88, 111, 117, 160, 165, 201

Cyst Degeneration, 163

depression, 26, 44, 100, 128, 142

detoxification, 43, 49, 72, 99, 118, 138, 159

detoxification pathways, 43, 72

DHA, 130

DHEAS, 159

dietary interventions, 167, 168

digestive health, 79, 80

EFT, 3, 8, 9, 21, 26, 27, 28, 29, 30, 31, 32, 33, 70, 158

Emotional Freedom Techniques, 8, 21, 26

endocrine system, 19, 35, 36, 37, 45, 146

endometriosis, 35, 37, 45, 120, 167

Endometriosis, 167

essential fatty acids, 98, 101, 130, 167

estrobolome, 101

estrogen, 34, 35, 36, 38, 39, 40, 41, 42, 43, 45, 46, 47, 64, 67, 69, 70, 72, 92, 93, 94, 95, 98, 99, 100, 101, 102, 117, 118, 119, 122, 124, 130, 133, 134, 137, 138, 139, 140, 141, 143, 155, 156, 157, 159, 212

estrogen balance, 119

estrogen dominance, 42, 43, 101, 138, 139

evening primrose oil, 130

fertility, 18, 36, 41, 44, 46, 53, 55, 56, 68, 78, 80, 81, 82, 83, 84, 98, 99, 100, 105, 108, 109, 119, 143, 148

Fiber, 101, 102

Fibroid Management, 167

fibroids, 128, 168

flax seeds, 95, 166

Flaxseed, 82, 83, 91, 92

Follicular Phase, 65, 67, 125

Functional Nutrition, 3, 8, 20, 21, 22, 23, 24, 27, 32, 33, 130, 205

gamma-linolenic acid, 98, 130

GLA, 98, 130

Gut Health, 101, 139, 141, 143

Hair Loss, 113

Hormonal Acne, 106, 117

hormonal balance, 19, 31, 37, 41, 45, 64, 65, 72, 78, 79, 87, 93, 98, 100, 103, 105, 106, 109, 117, 120, 124, 125, 128, 130, 133, 136, 139, 140, 141, 142, 143, 144, 145, 146, 147, 148, 149, 157, 159, 167, 168, 189, 191, 193, 211

hormones, 19, 30, 31, 32, 34, 35, 36, 37, 39, 40, 41, 42, 45, 48, 62, 63, 72, 74, 79, 87, 88, 96, 108, 116, 118, 119, 122, 128, 137, 140, 141, 142, 145, 147, 154, 156, 165, 176, 177, 210

infertility, 45, 119, 120

inflammation, 40, 65, 83, 85, 92, 97, 112, 117, 120, 130, 134, 145, 162, 166, 167, 168

Inflammation, 166

insulin, 36, 97, 110, 112, 138, 162, 166, 168

intermittent fasting, 67

Iron, 64, 102

libido, 40, 41, 68, 128, 142

lignans, 92, 95, 99, 100, 101, 119, 120, 124, 130, 134, 143

liver function, 43, 69, 98, 99

lunar, 52, 55, 56, 57, 58, 73, 74, 123, 124, 125, 160

233

Lunar, 124, 125, 144, 159

luteal phase, 39, 61, 62, 69, 70, 71, 72, 73, 75, 92, 95, 97, 98, 118, 123, 129, 130, 149

magnesium, 64, 92, 96, 97, 101, 102, 103, 104, 129, 132, 139, 143, 159, 171

menarche, 41, 76

menopause, 27, 31, 38, 39, 40, 41, 73, 79, 82, 95, 103, 118, 122, 127, 134, 151, 152, 155, 156, 157, 158, 159, 160

Menopause, 73, 151, 155, 156, 157, 158, 159, 229

menstrual cramps, 65, 97, 100

menstrual cycle, 35, 36, 37, 38, 39, 41, 42, 52, 53, 55, 57, 58, 61, 62, 63, 68, 70, 71, 72, 73, 78, 81, 87, 96, 98, 106, 107, 108, 111, 116, 118, 119, 121, 122, 125, 128, 131, 133, 136, 137, 142, 143, 144, 146, 147, 148, 149, 179, 180, 181, 182

Microbiome, 139

Moon, 50, 55, 56, 65, 76, 122, 124, 125, 159, 201, 215

moon phases, 57, 58, 73, 133, 134, 144, 149, 160

naturopath, 78

Nutritional Deficiencies, 139

nutritionist, 22, 202

Omega-3 fatty acids, 16, 65, 80, 92, 97, 118, 119, 120, 124, 130, 166, 175

Omega-6 fatty acids, 117, 124

ovarian, 35, 44, 81, 98, 100, 120, 163, 166

ovulation, 41, 44, 62, 63, 66, 67, 68, 69, 70, 72, 75, 87, 88, 92, 95, 96, 97, 107, 109, 110, 111, 119, 130, 131, 132, 137, 145, 147, 148

oxidative stress, 92, 159

PCOS, 35, 37, 44, 45, 97, 104, 110, 112, 119, 146, 162, 163, 165, 166, 168, 230

perimenopause, 39, 41, 118, 156

phytoestrogens, 93, 94, 117, 119, 130, 166, 167

PMS, 34, 64, 74, 78, 81, 87, 95, 99, 100, 101, 117, 130, 134, 136, 137, 138, 139, 140, 141, 142, 146, 148, 149, 189, 202, 225

polycystic ovary syndrome, 37, 104

post-menopause, 39

Postpartum, 127, 128

premenstrual syndrome, 117

probiotics, 16, 112, 141

progesterone, 34, 35, 36, 39, 40, 41, 42, 43, 44, 45, 67, 70, 72, 95, 96, 97, 98, 102, 110, 113, 117, 118, 119, 127, 130, 132, 137, 138, 139, 140, 141, 143, 145, 155, 159

prolactin, 41, 127

Puberty, 146, 201

pumpkin seeds, 64, 65, 82, 83, 84, 96, 97, 102, 123, 131, 159, 160, 168, 183

Recipes, 126, 170, 171, 175, 200, 233

Red Tent, 50, 51, 52, 54, 213

Seed Cycling, 3, 64, 78, 81, 82, 87, 90, 95, 97, 99, 101, 104, 105, 112, 116, 117, 119, 121, 122, 123, 125, 126, 127, 128, 129, 130, 135, 136, 140, 142, 143, 144, 145, 148, 151, 158, 159, 162, 166, 167, 168, 170, 171, 181, 196, 197, 200, 218, 220, 223, 225, 229, 230, 233

Seeds, 3, 5, 79, 80, 82, 83, 84, 85, 96, 97, 98, 99, 100, 103, 122, 124, 125, 133, 143, 159, 163, 168, 175, 187

Selenium, 98, 99, 102

serotonin, 72, 133

Sesame, 79, 84, 85, 99, 100, 101, 102, 122, 124, 125, 134, 159

sex hormone-binding globulin, 93, 94, 159

SHBG, 93, 159

sisterhood, 5, 33, 50, 52, 58, 154, 155

Sisterhood, 3, 5, 50, 213

sleep, 31, 45, 71, 97, 109, 112, 128, 133, 138, 145, 156, 158, 159

stress management, 105, 109

Sunflower, 80, 85, 86, 98, 99, 102, 122, 124, 125, 134, 159

sunflower seeds, 82, 85, 98, 99, 102, 123, 129, 159, 160, 168

Tapping, 3, 8, 26, 27, 30, 70, 123, 158

Teens, 136, 146, 147, 148, 225

testosterone, 34, 35, 40, 41, 110, 134

thyroid, 36, 42, 44, 98, 99, 102, 141, 159, 168

Thyroid, 42, 163, 168

thyroid health, 98, 99, 102, 159

vitamin B6, 64, 99, 100

vitamin D, 71, 139

Vitamin E, 98, 99, 102, 103, 117, 124, 159

weight management, 25, 118, 157, 158, 163

zinc, 96, 97, 99, 101, 103, 104, 117, 129, 132, 134, 143, 159, 168

www.ingramcontent.com/pod-product-compliance
Lightning Source LLC
Chambersburg PA
CBHW031316160426
43196CB00007B/554